Pathways to a Nursing Education Career:

Educating the Next Generation of Nurses

Judith A. Halstead, PhD, RN, ANEF, is Professor and Executive Associate Dean for Academic Affairs at Indiana University School of Nursing, Indianapolis. Prior to beginning her career in nursing education, Dr. Halstead served as a staff nurse in both university and private hospitals, specializing in oncology nursing. Her first appointment in nursing academe was as Instructor at Deaconess Hospital School of Nursing in Evansville, Indiana, and from there she moved to Indiana University School of Nursing and the University of Southern Indiana and back to Indiana University School of Nursing, where she has been Executive Associate Dean since 2004. Dr. Halstead currently teaches online graduate courses in nursing education. In her role as Executive Associate Dean, Dr. Halstead is responsible for providing leadership in curriculum planning, implementation, and evaluation of undergraduate and graduate nursing programs for Indiana University School of Nursing core school campuses of Indianapolis, Bloomington, and Columbus. She has delivered more than 50 national and international presentations and has been awarded over 4 million dollars in education and program grants. She is well published in refereed journals with 16 book chapters and 4 authored books, including the upcoming 4th edition of the leading comprehensive nurse educator text by Billings and Halstead, *Teaching in Nursing: A Guide for Faculty* (Saunders Elsevier). She is currently the president-elect of the National League for Nursing (2009–2011) and will assume the role of president 2011–2013.

Betsy Frank, PhD, RN, ANEF, is a professor at Indiana State University in the nursing program in the College of Nursing, Health, and Human Services (since 1998) where she was hired as Associate Professor in 1994. She has taught nursing since 1970 at a variety of programs in Ohio, New Mexico, and Texas. Her early clinical experience was in medical-surgical nursing. Her current teaching responsibilities include teaching in the online RN-BS and LPN-BS programs as well as in the University Honors Program and the graduate program in nursing administration. Dr. Frank has been awarded 6 grants, has delivered more than 20 professional presentations, has published many articles, has served as manuscript and book reviewer for nearly all nursing publishers, and has contributed chapters to numerous books, including three chapters for Feldman & Greenberg's (2005) *Educating Nurses for Leadership* (Springer Publishing Company), Oermann's *Annual Review of Nursing Education, Volume 6* (Springer Publishing Company), and several editions of Billings and Halstead's *Teaching in Nursing.*

Pathways to a Nursing Education Career:

Educating the Next Generation of Nurses

Judith A. Halstead, PhD, RN, ANEF
Betsy Frank, PhD, RN, ANEF

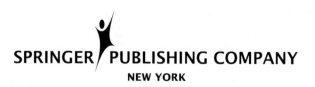

SPRINGER PUBLISHING COMPANY
NEW YORK

Springer Publishing Company, LLC
11 West 42nd Street
New York, NY 10036
www.springerpub.com

Acquisitions Editor: Margaret Zuccarini
Senior Editor: Rose Mary Piscitelli
Cover design: Steven Pisano
Project Manager: Nandini Loganathan
Composition: S4Carlisle Publishing Services

ISBN: 978-0-8261-0653-7
E-book ISBN: 978-0-8261-0654-4

10 11 12 13/ 5 4 3 2 1

Library of Congress Cataloging-in-Publication Data

Halstead, Judith A.
    Pathways to a nursing education career / Judith A. Halstead, Betsy Frank.
        p. ; cm.
    Includes bibliographical references.
    ISBN 978-0-8261-0653-7
 1. Nursing schools—Faculty.   I. Frank, Betsy. II. Title.
    [DNLM: 1. Faculty, Nursing.   2. Career Mobility.   3. Education, Nursing—methods. WY 19]
    RT90.H35 2011
    610.73071′1—dc22
                                                                        2010032940

Printed in the United States of America by Gasch Printing

Contents

Foreword

The shortage of nurse educators continues to be a problem, affecting the number of applicants who can be admitted by schools of nursing because of a lack of faculty to teach them. Many reports have documented the seriousness of the faculty shortage, which is projected to worsen; considering that the average age of nursing faculty is in the mid-50s, there will be a wave of retirements in the next 10 years combined with an inadequate number of new educators to fill those roles. One positive effect of this shortage, however, is the renewed interest in nursing education and growth of programs that prepare nurse educators. The awareness of the need for faculty, combined with the reality of current and projected faculty retirements, has led to the development and expansion of programs to prepare nurse educators. There also are mechanisms available such as loan repayment programs to support graduate students and nursing faculty who continue their education and make a commitment to remain in a faculty role.

Nursing education programs prepare new educators with knowledge and skills for effective teaching. However, gaining those competencies is not enough; nursing faculty need guidance and support for transitioning into their new roles and for developing their career as a nurse educator. This book was prepared for the novice nurse educator or graduate student beginning a career as a nursing faculty member. All too often novice educators enter their first teaching position and find their adjustment to the role of a faculty member daunting. While they have the essential competencies for teaching, they are unsure of their role in the school of nursing and how to resolve that uncertainty. They need a resource to turn to for understanding the educational institution, their role in it, and the expectations of the setting and administrator to whom they report. The beginning chapters of *Pathways to a Nursing Education Career* are a "must read" for any

novice educator transitioning from the role of clinician or graduate
student to educator. In those chapters, you will learn how to *become* a
faculty member, integrating the competencies you bring to the setting
with your new role as educator.

For a successful career as a nurse educator, it is important to
select the "right" school in which to teach, a school that reflects your
own values and is consistent with your personal and professional
goals. Strategies for assessing the school of nursing, its mission, environment, and expectations, and deciding if that is the best place to
begin one's career are presented in another chapter in the book.
This chapter will enable you to screen potential schools in which to
teach and make an informed decision about possible schools before
applying. You may have a lot of experience interviewing for clinical
or administrative positions in health systems, but if you have never
interviewed for a faculty position, it is a different process. For that
reason you will find guidelines for interviewing and other areas to
assess when making this important decision about where to teach.

Teaching can be stressful for the educator, both novice and experienced. First, it is time-consuming, and preparing for teaching activities takes longer when one is inexperienced. This time commitment
may create added stress for faculty members who also are involved in
writing grant proposals, conducting research, writing for publication,
serving on committees, and maintaining a clinical practice as part
of their role. Balancing these multiple roles, all of which take time,
can be stressful for both beginning and experienced nursing faculty.
Strategies for coping with these stresses and demands; adjusting to
the role of the faculty member; and finding time for family, friends,
and self are described in a chapter in this book.

Other chapters explain components of the faculty role that novice
educators and new graduates may not understand. There is a chapter
on the role of the faculty member as scholar. In that chapter, you will
learn about varied models of scholarship used in schools of nursing,
how to assess the definition of scholarship in your own institution,
and strategies for setting career goals for your own scholarship. You
will also learn about resources you can use for your own scholarly
work. There is another chapter that explains the service commitment
of nursing faculty and what that means in your career development.

Teaching is an interpersonal process: Students learn through their
interactions with the teacher in a caring and supportive environment.
Because of the importance of this relationship, one of the chapters

in the book is devoted to preparing you for interacting with students as part of your teaching role. This chapter has other critical information in it, for example, for understanding the teaching workload in a school of nursing and organizations to develop your role as a nurse educator, among others.

The eighth chapter in the book provides valuable information for your career development as a nursing faculty. Too often educators, and other professionals as well, do not reflect on their career goals and where they want to be 5 and 10 years from when they started their roles as faculty. This chapter is valuable because it will help you to learn not only about promotion and tenure in different schools of nursing, other requirements for nursing faculty, and portfolio development, but also about strategies to plan for professional growth and map out a career trajectory.

Many texts are available on curriculum development, teaching, assessment, evaluation, and other areas to provide the knowledge and skills essential for the nurse educator. However, these texts do not prepare the educator for transitioning into the role or for career development. *Pathways to a Nursing Education Career* is an outstanding resource for the novice nurse educator, and this easy-to-read book provides resources for new faculty members to transition successfully into an academic educator role and continue their career development.

Marilyn H. Oermann, PhD, RN, FAAN, ANEF
Professor and Division Chair, School of Nursing
University of North Carolina at Chapel Hill
Chapel Hill, North Carolina

Preface

If you are in nursing education courses in your graduate program or if you are a new nursing faculty member or considering an academic career, this book is for you. With the current shortage of nursing faculty, many nurses in clinical practice will be making the transition to the role of nurse educator. Making this transition requires forethought, education, and support. We anticipate this book will help you as you make that transition. Although targeted at novice educators and graduate students, we anticipate that you will return to this book during your career when you need support as you undertake the successes and challenges of what we hope will be a long and rewarding career in nursing education. Beginning nurse educators who teach in any setting—community colleges, liberal arts colleges, comprehensive universities, or research universities—will find this book useful. With the focus on novice nurse educators, faculty who teach graduate courses in nursing education will want to use this text as a course resource.

The transition from a practice role to a faculty role can be overwhelming, especially in the first year of being in a faculty role. Therefore, each chapter in this book has real-life advice aimed at smoothing that transition. Based on our expertise and experiences, the chapters focus upon how to develop in one's nurse educator role. We do not provide a comprehensive discussion about curriculum development, evaluation, or teaching strategies. Rather, we discuss issues related to role development as a nurse educator.

Chapter 1 sets the stage for faculty role development. We provide an overview of issues and trends affecting the nursing faculty shortage.

In Chapter 2, you learn what is involved in assuming the nursing faculty role. We introduce you to the National League for Nursing's Core Competencies of Nurse Educators (2005). These competencies will serve as your guide as you develop into your role as a nursing faculty member.

In Chapter 3, you learn about the job interview process. We present examples of interview questions that prospective employers might ask you, as well as questions that you might ask employers. One critical facet of the job search is determining which type of institution best matches your career goals. We provide questions to help you think about whether you want to focus on things like teaching or research or some combination thereof.

Chapter 4 presents a discussion of the tripartite mission for nursing faculty. You will learn about what factors to consider when trying to balance all aspects of your role with your personal life. Balancing your life is as critical to your success in the nurse educator role as is building your support network. You will learn strategies for bringing balance to your life and acquiring a professional network of colleagues. Knowing about policies and procedures is also a part of your orientation to the faculty role. Therefore, we provide a discussion about policies and procedures common to all academic institutions.

Chapters 5, 6, and 7 supply a detailed discussion of each of the components of your faculty role. Chapter 5 discusses the teaching role in detail. We present facets of the teaching role including how institutions determine faculty teaching assignments.

In Chapter 6, we present a discussion about developing as a scholar in your faculty role. All components of the Boyer model of scholarship are presented. You will learn how various academic institutions envision the scholarship component of the faculty role.

The service component is presented in Chapter 7. Within this chapter are descriptions of academic, professional, and community service. Service at the local, regional, state, and national levels is discussed. Networking as a strategy for engaging in professional service is stressed.

Transitioning into the faculty role is just the beginning of your career. Therefore, Chapter 8 presents strategies for short- and long-term career planning. You will learn how to prepare a dossier for retention, tenure, and promotion. Regardless of whether you are in a traditional or clinical tenure track appointment or on a multiyear or year-to-year contract, preparing a portfolio that accurately portrays your accomplishments is essential. Surviving reappointment and gaining tenure are just part of your career success. You will reflect on long-term goals that guide your career development. You will also learn about the importance of mentors in advancing your career.

Finally, in Chapter 9, the Afterword, we share our stories. These stories have set the stage for this book.

Each chapter includes exhibits that summarize important information and case studies that faculty can use in graduate nursing education courses and in planning new faculty orientation programs. Faculty teaching courses for prospective nurse educators can also use the reflective questions, called "Think About" (placed within the text), and the "Opportunities for Further Reflection" (at the end of each chapter) to help students consider how the material is relevant to them. Faculty in their first few years as educators may also want to return to some of these exhibits as needed.

In the Appendix, we have provided a list of printed and Web-based resources that students and novice faculty can draw upon as they transition to a faculty role. These resources (e.g., where to find good places that provide faculty development opportunities and provide a forum for you to present your scholarship) will help you develop into a faculty role.

We wish to acknowledge Margaret Zuccarini and Elizabeth Stump. They, like us, believe that this book will serve as a great resource for new nurse educators.

We would also like to thank our families for all their support throughout our careers. Judy would like to thank her husband, Jerry, and her children, David and Angela. Betsy would like to thank her husband, Dick, and her children, Becki and Laurel. Without their encouragement, this book would not have been possible.

Judith A. Halstead
Betsy Frank

Pathways to a Nursing Education Career:

Educating the Next Generation of Nurses

Chapter 1

The Nursing Faculty Role: Issues and Trends

Readers of this book will likely fall into two primary groups of individuals—those who are aspiring to a nursing faculty role or those who have already accepted their first academic teaching position and are new to the faculty role. Regardless of your personal situation, congratulations upon contemplating and accepting the opportunities and challenges a career in academia will bring to you. You are embarking upon a career path that will provide you with a multitude of professional and personal rewards.

As an aging workforce of nursing faculty prepare to retire, the nursing profession is experiencing a time when the numbers of faculty—those who are charged with preparing our next generation of nurses—are reaching a level of critical shortage. Our profession is in great need of academically and experientially qualified educators to replace those who are retiring within the next 10 years. Those who are retiring may continue, on a part-time basis, to provide quality educational experiences for our students. However, those who work part-time will more than likely not be available to do the necessary committee work and student advising. Given the current and anticipated nursing shortage, the need for new full-time faculty to increase the number of new nursing graduates is great.

Many of these new faculty will be expert clinicians but inexperienced as teachers in the classroom and clinical settings. For most, it will be their first exposure to the tripartite role expectations of teaching, research, and service that are typically associated with being a faculty member. As a new or aspiring academician, you probably find yourself with a number of questions about how to best develop your career in academia to meet the expectations of the faculty role.

In addition to the more traditional expectations associated with the faculty role, there are emerging issues and trends in academia and practice that will influence and impact the future roles of nursing

1

faculty. The health care setting is an increasingly complex and chaotic environment in which to practice and instruct students. Similarly, educational environments are experiencing declining resource allocations at the same time that public expectations regarding performance outcomes are increasing. The purpose of this chapter is to explore issues and trends associated with the nursing faculty role so that you are able to understand the full context of the role and how it is influenced by internal and external environmental factors. The nursing and nurse faculty shortage, increasing complexity of the health care system, changing dynamics in higher education, integration of technology into education and health care, and increasing need for collaborations and partnerships to provide quality education health care are some of the major trends that are currently affecting the role of nursing faculty.

THE NURSING AND NURSE FACULTY SHORTAGE

The nursing workforce in the United States is on the verge of one of the most significant nursing shortages our country has ever experienced in modern times. The economic recession that began in the latter part of this decade has slowed the rise in nursing shortage numbers due to nurses either choosing to postpone retirement or returning to the workforce. However, this is considered to be only a temporary abatement of the impending shortage. It has been estimated that by the year 2025 the U.S. health care system will have a shortage of approximately 260,000 nurses (Buerhaus, Auerbach, & Staiger, 2009). The primary reason for the projected shortage of nurses is the aging of the nursing workforce leading to large numbers of retirements. However, it must be acknowledged that nurses also leave the profession due to dissatisfaction with the work environment, thus compounding the shortage issue.

At the same time that a nursing workforce shortage is being projected, the health care sector is continuing to grow in all arenas, including acute care, long-term care, and ambulatory care settings (American Association of Colleges of Nursing, 2008, 2009). This growth in the health care sector will provide additional employment opportunities for registered nurses. Skilled long-term care settings have an especially acute need for increasing the numbers of registered nurses employed. In addition, with health care reform being aggressively pursued by legislators and health care providers, additional workforce demands for registered nurses and advanced practice nurses will likely emerge, especially in the primary health care environments. Health care reform will also demand that nurses demonstrate a different set of competencies with a focus on interdisciplinary, evidence-based, patient-centered care that is delivered with the intent to provide a seamless transition in the health care that is provided across the health care continuum.

Another factor related to the nursing shortage that must be considered in this discussion is the educational preparation of nurses who are in the workforce. The majority of the nursing workforce providing direct patient care is initially prepared at the associate degree level. These nurses provide safe and competent patient care, yet additional educational preparation is necessary to acquire the systems-level knowledge and leadership skills required to function in unstructured, chaotic work environments. To meet the demands of an increasingly complex health care environment, as well as the need for advanced practice nurses, nurse researchers, and nurse educators, we must begin to prepare more nurses with baccalaureate and graduate nursing degrees.

The Health Resources and Services Administration (2010) reported in its 2008 survey of registered nurses that only 36.8% of registered nurses held a baccalaureate degree and 13.2% of registered nurses held advanced nursing degrees at the master's or doctoral level. These numbers suggest that the nursing workforce is not well positioned at this time to strategically participate in and lead efforts to reform health care to meet the health care needs of Americans. It is essential that the academic progression of nurses be facilitated to produce the numbers of registered nurses with advanced education that are projected to be needed in the workforce. In 2010, the Tri-Council for Nursing (consisting of the American Association of Colleges of Nursing, American Nurses Association, American Organization of Nurse Executives, and the National League for Nursing) issued a consensus policy statement, which calls for strategies facilitating the educational advancement of nurses to prepare a better educated nursing workforce.

Because of the projected nursing shortage, there is tremendous pressure on academic institutions to admit more nursing students and increase the numbers of graduates. This increased pressure comes at a time when we are also experiencing a shortage of qualified faculty. Our nursing programs are at capacity in large part due to the lack of qualified faculty. With the average age of nursing faculty hovering in the mid-50s, there will be large numbers of faculty retirements within the next few years. Noncompetitive faculty salaries, as compared to positions in the practice setting, deter some nurses from considering a career in an academic setting and thus make recruitment of faculty difficult.

The lack of academically and experientially qualified faculty to take the place of retiring faculty will strain the resources of our academic workforce for the foreseeable future. Coupled with the nursing faculty shortage is the shortage of qualified academic administrators in our nursing programs. Inexperienced faculty will require mentoring in the classroom and clinical settings; inexperienced academic administrators will likewise require mentoring to effectively lead nursing education programs.

The discipline of nursing is also being affected by the lack of nursing education researchers and the lack of rigorous, funded nursing education research, especially in the area of how best to teach nursing students in the clinical setting. For the past two decades in the nursing profession, preparing nursing faculty who were experts in nursing education research and the scholarship of teaching has been considered to be of secondary importance to preparing nurses as experts in clinical nursing research. This necessary emphasis on developing nursing's expertise in clinical research led to a paucity of nursing education research, with few funds being allocated to support educational research. Recently, the need to apply an evidence-based approach to our teaching has been called for by the profession, and a renewed interest in nursing education research has developed along with calls for increased funding of the research (National League for Nursing [NLN], 2007). We will need more nursing faculty with the skills necessary to pursue educational research as a viable research career and add to the science of nursing education.

Therefore, how does the nursing and faculty shortage affect you in your role as a nurse educator? You have chosen an exciting and challenging time to become a nursing faculty—we are experiencing fundamental shifts in how we approach the "business" of nursing education. The nursing shortage requires us to consider innovative means by which to prepare safe, competent nurses in numbers adequate enough to meet the workforce demand. We are also being asked to consider ways to accelerate the preparation of nurses with advanced nursing degrees to meet the needs for advanced clinicians, researchers, and educators. As a new nurse educator, you will have the opportunity to respond to these needs and create new models by which we will educate our students.

The nursing profession must address how to attract new faculty and prepare them for the role. The lack of experienced faculty means that faculty development programs will become even more essential to help novice faculty develop the competencies associated with the nurse educator role (NLN, 2005). The development of academic leaders in nursing is another critical need. Although the nursing and faculty shortages do provide us with many challenges, the opportunities to create a long-term, rewarding career in nursing education and to impact the future of the nursing profession by designing new education models are endless for those who choose nursing education as a career path. Nurses who become nursing faculty at this time will personally benefit from the profession's reaffirmation of the importance of preparing the next generation of nursing faculty and the renewed attention to nursing education research and scholarship.

Think About . . .

What is the status of available nursing faculty positions in your region? What are the major challenges facing nursing faculty? How are nursing programs responding to these challenges?

CHANGES IN THE HEALTH CARE SYSTEM

It is no secret that the health care system in the United States has become increasingly complex. Critics are calling for reform to ensure that the health care needs of citizens are met. If you are transitioning from the practice setting into education, you are very familiar with the challenges facing nurses in the health care environment. Your new challenge as an educator will be to apply your current knowledge of clinical practice in the health care system to developing learning experiences for your students, which will provide them with the competencies required to practice in such a setting.

The Institute of Medicine (IOM, 2003) identified five key competencies that all health care professionals needed for practice in the 21st century: an emphasis on patient-centered care, informatics, quality improvement, evidence-based practice, and interprofessional team work.

The IOM further called for educational reform and the creation of clinical education models that would enable students to achieve these competencies. At the same time, creating a health care culture that promotes patient safety is another high-priority need that has been identified. Health care reform will likely increase the need for advanced practice nurses who have specialized in primary care and nurses who understand transitional models of health care. The use of health care technology calls for health care professionals to be savvy users of the technology while understanding the legal and ethical implications of technology for the delivery of patient care. The competencies required of health care professionals to deliver safe, quality care will continue to be debated by leaders in health care and health care education. No one can anticipate all the changes in health care delivery that will occur. Therefore, educators will need to prepare future practitioners to cope with this rapidly changing health care environment. More important than teaching psychomotor skills will be the ability to help students think critically and apply what they know to new situations.

Such calls for changes in how we deliver health care and practice nursing have direct implications for you in your role as a nurse educator. First, these changes require us to closely examine our curriculum and revise our current models of clinical nursing education. There is no predetermined "blueprint" for what these curricular revisions should look like; in many ways, we are moving into a future where it is difficult to predict what educational models will be most effective for producing the desired outcome for practice. We will need nurse educators who are willing to challenge the status quo and risk change and innovation to produce new curriculum models.

Second, we will need nursing faculty who are competent in evidence-based practice, informatics, quality improvement, interprofessional teamwork, and patient-centered care that is delivered with a focus on a culture of safety. Faculty will need to understand new models of health care delivery and be competent with the use of health care technology. Ongoing faculty development will be essential. For some of us, this may mean returning to school or taking continuing education courses to maintain our competence or develop new skills.

The implication for you as a novice nurse educator is to understand that the relationship between practice and education is a dynamic one. The rapidity with which the health care environment is changing creates challenges for nursing faculty who struggle to keep curriculum relevant. Because of this dynamic relationship, it is essential that education and practice work closely together to develop curricula that produce graduates with the requisite competencies. This also means that you are entering nursing education as a career at a time when our traditional "means" of delivering curriculum are being questioned, some may even say challenged, with an urgency with which they have never been questioned before in order to meet the needs of health care reform. Being comfortable with ambiguity and change will be important attributes for you to have as a nurse educator.

Think About . . .

What additional health care delivery changes can you identify that could have an impact on your role as a nurse educator in an academic setting? What are some means by which you can stay abreast of health care trends in your new role?

TRENDS IN HIGHER EDUCATION

Regardless of the type of institution in which you choose to work as a nursing faculty, your role will be closely affected by trends in higher education. If you are transitioning from the practice setting, some of these issues in all likelihood will be new to you; others, such as managing shrinking resources and demonstrating outcomes, will seem very familiar albeit in a different environmental context. Similar to the changes that are occurring in health care and affecting nursing practice, the changing dynamics in higher education will affect the future role of faculty in ways that are likely not yet fully understood by members of the academy.

Arguably the most significant trend currently facing higher education is the economic conditions that many institutions find themselves facing—shrinking resources from the state (for public state-supported institutions), caps placed on rising tuition costs and fees, endowment funds that have declined significantly, aging physical facilities that demand repair, and rising costs for employee benefits (e.g., health care insurance). In many cases, these conditions have combined to create the "perfect storm" for colleges and institutions throughout the United States, causing the institutions to resort to a variety of strategies to preserve their financial status and remain solvent. Some of these strategies include hiring and wage freezes, reduction of staff and faculty through layoffs and attrition, mandatory furlough of employees to conserve cash flow, elimination of academic programs with low enrollments, elimination of travel and development funds for faculty, and restrictions on general spending.

At the same time that institutions are grappling with financial crises, recruiting and retaining the "best and the brightest" faculty remains a source of chief concern, as faculty are the lifeblood of the educational environment. In order to deal with current and future realities in funding limitations, you can anticipate that institutions will consider innovative ways to attract and retain faculty even in the face of economic downturns. For example, institutions will seek means by which they can reward faculty for excellence even when wages remain frozen.

Without the intellectual capital of faculty, the institutions would not be able to produce their "product"—graduates who are well educated and prepared to enter the workforce. For nursing faculty, the current economic realities mean that they are facing larger class sizes due to fewer faculty, salaries that are frozen and falling further behind their colleagues in practice, and an expectation that they conduct their "business" differently in the future to accommodate the lack of available resources. Creativity and flexibility will certainly be two qualities required of all nursing faculty to meet these challenges and preserve program quality. For those faculty who embrace change and are not rooted in doing things "the way they have always been done," these times can be looked upon as times of opportunity to investigate new models of teaching nursing.

Even with shrinking resources, or maybe *because* of shrinking resources, institutions of higher education are under closer public scrutiny. Institutions of higher learning are being held accountable for demonstrating performance outcomes that are deemed acceptable by external constituents. State legislatures, in particular, are closely examining the educational outcomes of institutions and, in some cases, allocating funds based on performance indicators that have been set by the legislature. Such performance indicators include measures such as student recruitment, retention, and graduation rates. Institutions that have high attrition rates or cannot graduate their students within a certain period of time (e.g., within 5–6 years for a 4-year degree) may find their state funding decreased until they demonstrate improvement in the key indicators. This trend of external scrutiny is only likely to increase, and higher education finds itself needing to examine and be accountable for practices that up until now have been its sole prerogative to set.

Various curriculum trends within higher education can also have an impact on the curriculum of nursing programs and thus the role of nursing faculty. For example, campus-level faculty councils set general education requirements within institutions. Periodically, these requirements go through a faculty-driven review process, which can result in changes in the requirements. Such changes can lead to a need to modify discipline-specific curriculum plans of study. Some current curriculum trends within higher education include the emphasis on civic engagement and service learning and the increasing influence of globalization on the educational experience. Many schools of nursing will need to include opportunities in their curricula for students to participate in civic engagement and international study in keeping with the parent institution's mission to provide these learning experiences to students.

Performance indicators that are set by external constituencies (i.e., accrediting bodies, state legislators) may require the campus-level collection of evaluation data from all faculty, which in turn has the potential to affect the teaching and evaluation strategies you use in your classroom. Case Study 1.1 illustrates a situation in which a new faculty member, David, realizes that to fully understand his new role as nursing faculty, he needs to also understand the higher education environment in which he is teaching.

Mirroring societal demographic changes, the increasing diversity of the student body in our institutions of higher education is a continuing trend that affects nursing faculty. In an effort to meet the needs of their region, many institutions have a mission to recruit students who have been previously underrepresented in the student body. The numbers of international students seeking a college education in the United States, including nursing, are also increasing. Meeting the learning needs of diverse students in classroom and clinical settings can be a complex endeavor. Faculty need to be increasingly knowledgeable about how learning can be affected by cultural differences, especially when teaching in the clinical setting where health beliefs, personal space, and communication can be heavily influenced by cultural values.

David: Nursing Education Issues and Trends

David has recently accepted a position as an assistant professor of nursing at a regional state-supported college. This is his first academic position in higher education. In his doctoral program, he did not have the opportunity to take any course work related to nursing education. He thought he was well prepared for a faculty role, having been exposed to a rigorous course of study in theory, research, and statistics at a well-respected university. However, in his first months in his new position, he noticed that in faculty meetings he really didn't understand the discussions that nursing faculty were having about the campus's newly proposed general education curriculum. How could college faculty who weren't even nurses influence the curriculum of the nursing program? In addition, he had received a request from his department chair to participate in collecting some student evaluation data from his courses that were supposed to measure the extent to which students were applying the campus's core concepts of undergraduate learning. He didn't realize that he was responsible for having students apply the core concepts in his course and didn't understand how the core concepts related to the critical care nursing concepts he was teaching. At one faculty meeting, the dean of the nursing program announced that state appropriations to the nursing program may be cut due to financial difficulties that the state was having and that these cuts could impact how faculty implemented the nursing curriculum. David began to understand that being a nursing expert in critical care was not sufficient to fully understand his role. He recognized that he needed to also understand the context of higher education and the many factors that could affect his teaching. Now, what could he do to develop a better understanding of the higher education environment?

These are just a few of the current trends in higher education that will have an impact on your work as a nursing faculty. New trends are ever emerging, and as a faculty in higher education you will be responsible for staying abreast of the issues and understanding the implications for your program and students.

Think About . . .

*How familiar are you with trends in higher education?
What are some ways by which you can become more
knowledgeable about higher education in your
local area, state, and nation?*

TRENDS IN NURSING EDUCATION

As in higher education, trends in nursing education will influence how you implement your role as a nurse educator. Developing flexible learning environments, trimming "overstuffed" curricula, addressing the need for new clinical education models, and preparing graduates with the competencies to practice in a reformed health care system are examples of current trends that nursing faculty are currently considering.

Learning environments are changing. Nursing faculty of the future will need to be competent in designing learning spaces that are "virtual" classrooms and made flexible to meet the needs of learners and facilitate active learning strategies. Courses will be less likely to be structured in the typical 16-week semester and more likely to be designed as "modules" that can be delivered in alternate time frames. Technology will continue to influence the delivery of nursing education, creating even greater access to education for the nursing workforce. The impact of technology is discussed at greater length in the section that follows.

As nursing curricula become more and more crowded with content, nursing faculty are grappling with the issue of what "should" be in the nursing curriculum. How do faculty decide what are essential learning experiences for nursing students? How do faculty decide what content should be included and what should be eliminated? Faculty will need to learn to teach more conceptually and with an emphasis on developing the clinical reasoning skills of students instead of focusing as much on "content."

Clinical nursing education models are being reexamined for effectiveness and efficiency in preparing students for practice in the "real world." There will be more emphasis on the learning triad of student–preceptor–faculty and how best to collaboratively partner in the delivery of clinical learning experiences for both undergraduate and graduate nursing students.

There will be a continued emphasis on facilitating the academic progression of nurses in the workforce. As stated previously, the nursing profession needs greater numbers of nurses prepared with graduate degrees to be advanced practice nurses, nursing administrators, and nurse educators. To respond to these needs, nursing faculty will be developing educational models that accelerate the academic progression of nurses.

Nursing faculty will also need to work collaboratively with their colleagues in practice to identify emerging practice needs that will come about as a result of health care reform. Faculty will need to keep curricula dynamic and be able to incorporate new competencies and skills as demanded by the evolving needs of the health care system.

THE IMPACT OF TECHNOLOGY

The integration of technology into health care and education has significant influence on your role as a nursing faculty and as such deserves to be discussed in a separate section. As you are already aware, health care is delivered in a technology-driven environment that contributes greatly to the complexity of the practice setting. Electronic health records, telehealth, e-ICUs, and a vast array of sophisticated patient care delivery devices and monitors are just a few examples of how reliant the health care system is on the use of technology.

The widespread use of health care technology requires that nurses continually update their knowledge and skill in the use of the technology. Legal and ethical issues, such as end-of-life support decisions and patient confidentiality concerns, are also significant, with the use of technology contributing to the many bioethical issues present in health care. As you transition from the practice setting to the academic setting it will still be essential, yet a challenge, for you to remain current with the technology used in practice. You will want to consider how you will remain current in the use of technology that is specific to your practice area.

At the same time you are considering how to remain technologically current in the practice setting, you will be asked to develop what will likely be new competencies in the use of educational, or instructional, technology. Technology has been fully integrated throughout the education environment, and it is not possible for faculty to teach without using it. In fact, students fully expect that faculty will be comfortable with the use of technology and may likely consider those faculty who do not use technology to be out of date and incompetent.

What types of technology will you use in your role as a faculty? For a start, for your own professional use you will need to be comfortable with the common software found on a desktop or laptop computer. Writing, presentation, and spreadsheet software programs will be provided to you by your institution. Software that helps you track reference notes and run statistical programs is also frequently supplied. Creating tables and formatting documents will be essential skills for you to develop. Using e-mail or other forms of electronic communication to communicate with your colleagues and students, and managing the volume of your e-mail, will be other skills for you to master. Although many of you may already have these skills, if you do not, begin to acquire them now, as the effective use of technology will be the backbone of your productivity as a faculty.

From an instructional perspective, your use of technology will vary considerably depending on the type of courses you teach. All faculty should master the use of presentation software (e.g., PowerPoint) for instructional purposes. However, learning how to create computer-generated presentations that use good instructional design principles and facilitate active learning in the classroom instead of passive listening will be important. The use of mobile devices, podcasts, vodcasts, personal response devices (commonly referred to as "clickers"), and computer-assisted media has a place in your instructional efforts depending on the learning outcomes you wish to achieve.

It is very common for faculty to be required to learn a Web-based course management system by which they can deliver their course materials, or even an entire course, to students. A course management system is a software program, provided and supported by your academic institution, that provides a common platform students can use to access course materials, take online tests, send e-mail messages to course faculty and classmates, and participate in discussion forums and chat rooms that facilitate dialogue about course content. Such systems can be used in combination with traditional face-to-face courses that meet in the classroom, or they can be used to deliver courses online in an asynchronous manner. If you are assigned to teach a distance-learning course that has synchronous class meeting times, you may be asked to learn how to teach using Web-based video-conferencing software that connects students at a distance via Web-cameras from their own home or office to you in your own office or classroom.

The use of simulation technology is a current trend in nursing education. Simulation technology can range from the use of static mannequins for mastering psychomotor skills to high-fidelity mannequins programmed to provide human-like responses to care delivered by students. The use of such technology, especially the high-fidelity models, requires significant institutional investment in faculty development and equipment. If this is a technology that would be meaningful to use in the courses you are assigned to teach, you can expect to devote time to developing your own competence with the use of the technology. "Virtual world" technology, which can be used to create virtual patient care learning scenarios, is another form of simulation technology emerging within nursing education that faculty are learning how to use in the curriculum.

As you can see, the use of technology in nursing education can take many different forms. Whether you are teaching in the practice setting or the educational setting, you can be assured that you will be interfacing with technology and will need to find methods by which you can feel competent in your use of it.

Think About . . .

How would you rate your current comfort level with the use of technology in the practice setting and the educational setting? What strategies might you use to increase your competence in using technology in your role as a nursing faculty?

THE IMPORTANCE OF PARTNERSHIPS

The formation of mutually beneficial partnerships is an essential element to functioning as a nursing faculty. Because of the complexity of the issues that we are facing in higher education, health care, and nursing education, and the scarcity of resources that we have to address the issues, collaborative partnerships are increasingly important to the success and sustainability of nursing programs. Such partnerships may involve nursing colleagues in academia, practice partners, interprofessional teams, or community partners. You can expect to be involved in a number of partnerships throughout the course of your academic career, and developing the collaborative "know-how" to work effectively with partners is a skill that will be highly valued.

Forming academic partnerships with other schools of nursing is one means by which programs can share and maximize resources. For example, regional or statewide collaboration agreements have been formed to teach common curricula across programs, to deliver faculty development programs around a centrally held interest, and to facilitate the implementation of graduate programs using faculty expertise from across the partner schools.

Academic–practice partnerships have become fairly common as well. Nursing education programs and health care agencies have found that, by working together to address challenges facing both, innovative and mutually beneficial solutions can be developed. For example, a number of partnerships have been formed to help offset the nursing faculty shortage. Clinical agencies may provide qualified staff to nursing programs to serve as faculty in exchange for the opportunity to recruit graduates from the program. Other partnerships feature the development of unique clinical models used to deliver undergraduate or graduate clinical education with the intent of improving student competencies. One such example is the development of dedicated education units in which students work one on one with a dedicated preceptor, immersing themselves in the work of the nurse. Joint appointments are another means of collaborating, allowing the expertise of selected individuals to be used in both settings. The goal of any academic–practice partnership is to use the expertise of those involved to the fullest extent possible, realizing that the combination of clinical expertise and educational expertise is most likely the best approach to identifying workable solutions to complex issues.

In response to numerous calls for interprofessional collaboration in the health professions to improve the safety and quality of patient care, interprofessional partnerships have become critical. The two nursing accrediting bodies, the Commission on Collegiate Nursing Education and the National League for Nursing Accrediting Commission, have standards that require programs to address the interdisciplinary learning experiences available within their curriculum. Partnerships may be formed to foster the integration of interdisciplinary educational experiences in the curriculum, to facilitate research, or to promote faculty development in teaching strategies (e.g., simulations, problem-based learning, etc.), to name just a few examples. Interprofessional collaborations may also occur in the academic setting when faculty from various disciplines come together to share common interests and collaborate on teaching and research projects.

Community partnerships are also essential to nursing programs. In some cases, the desire to establish community partnerships goes beyond the need to provide clinical learning experiences for students. The educational institution may have as part of its mission the goal of establishing partnerships with the surrounding community to facilitate positive "town–gown" relationships. Civic engagement and service learning can also be important aspects of the institution's mission. Civic engagement and service learning, as examples of community partnerships, are discussed in more depth in Chapter 7.

In your faculty role, you can be expected to participate in partnerships that will require you to develop skills related to communication, negotiation, collegiality, collaboration, and mutual trust and respect. You can also capitalize on relationships that you have already developed through your experience in the practice setting. Although it is true that in academia you are most often rewarded for the accomplishments you achieve on your own, the ability to form and nurture partnerships is becoming increasingly important in academia and a highly valuable skill for faculty to possess.

Think About . . .

What professional partnerships have you participated in previously? What skills did you develop in those partnerships that you can transfer to the academic setting?

THE FUTURE OF THE NURSING FACULTY ROLE

As you can tell from this brief discussion of issues and trends influencing nursing education, your faculty role is affected by many forces internal and external to the nursing profession. Although the number of challenges facing nursing education may appear to be overwhelming to some degree, this is actually a wonderful time to invest in an academic career as a nurse educator. The need for new educators with new ideas about how to best prepare future nurses is critical. For those nurses who relish the invitation to be creative and shape the future of the nursing profession through shaping its educational models, there has never been a more opportune time to do so.

National policy makers and funding agencies recognize the importance of health profession education. Nurses are in the forefront to take advantage of this new respect for education. As faculty, nurses have long been among some of the most respected educators on our campuses of higher education. There is a need for educational research that demonstrates how education impacts the quality of patient care and how to most effectively educate health professionals so that they acquire the necessary competencies for contemporary practice. Once again, nurse faculty are in a leadership position among health care professionals to contribute significantly to the educational research agenda in the health professions.

It is our opinion that the future of nursing education is indeed bright. An academic career in nursing education is a very rewarding career to have—in what other position can you influence the future professional practice of so many nurses, especially as their initial professional identities and values are being formed? The benefits of a career as a nursing faculty are many. The rest of the chapters in this book will guide you along the pathway of starting such a career.

Opportunities for Further Reflection

1. Consider your geographic region and the forces that are affecting nursing education and the faculty role. Are the forces comparable to those that you read about in this chapter? Are there additional forces to consider?

REFERENCES

American Association of Colleges of Nursing. (2008). *2007–2008 Enrollment and graduations in baccalaureate and graduate programs in nursing.* Washington, DC: Author.

American Association of Colleges of Nursing. (2009). *Nursing shortage fact sheet* (updated September 2009). Retrieved June 13, 2010, from http://www.aacn.nche.edu/media/FactSheets/NursingShortage.htm

Buerhaus, P., Auerbach, D., & Staiger, D. (2009). The recent surge in nurse employment: Causes and implications. *Health Affairs, 28*(4), 657–668.

Health Resources and Services Administration. (2010, March). *The registered nurse population: Findings from the March 2008 National Sample Survey of Registered Nurses.* Washington, DC: U.S. Department of Health and Human Services. Retrieved August 21, 2010, from http://bhpr.hrsa.gov/healthworkforce/rnsurvey/initialfindings2008.pdf

Institute of Medicine. (2003). *Health professions education: A bridge to quality.* Washington, DC: The National Academies Press.

National League for Nursing. (2005). *Core competencies of nurse educators.* Retrieved June 13, 2010, from http://www.nln.org/facultydevelopment/pdf/corecompetencies.pdf

National League for Nursing. (2007). *The need for funding for nursing education research.* Retrieved June 13, 2010, from http://www.nln.org/aboutnln/PositionStatements/nursingedresearch_051807.pdf

Tri-Council for Nursing. (2010). *Educational advancement of registered nurses: A consensus position.* Retrieved June 13, 2010, from http://www.nln.org/newsreleases/tri-council.pdf

Assuming the Faculty Role

Accepting a faculty position and assuming the faculty role is professionally transforming in many respects. Depending on the type of clinical position you have held, if you are transitioning from a clinical position, you are probably accustomed to working in a rapidly paced environment with more or less defined work hours. Providing direct patient care requires that every minute of your workday be focused on delivering the safest care possible and anticipating the needs of your patients, often making clinical decisions in split seconds that can dramatically alter patient care outcomes. There is little time for on-the-job reflection about your practice or for review of the latest literature. If you are transitioning from a graduate student role to a faculty role, you have probably become accustomed to working primarily on your own to complete learning assignments that have clearly assigned due dates. The reward system is relatively immediate—submitted course assignments will yield a course grade, so you quickly become aware of the outcomes related to your work.

Academia is different. Although the faculty role can vary significantly depending on the type of academic institution by which you are employed, there are certain commonalities associated with the role that are independent of institutional context. The hours and activities of the faculty workweek are often flexible and highly variable, encompassing teaching, service, scholarship, and practice—frequently all within the same week. On-the-job evaluation and reflection are key components of the faculty role, as is immersion in the literature to remain current. The responsibilities associated with the demands of the faculty role are multidimensional and require you to be able to conceptualize as well as operationalize projects. The pace of the academic environment does not carry with it the same sense of urgency that a patient care environment does. Certainly, deadlines are set and must be met, but the critical elements of the role that are expected—such as your course preparation for teaching; your research and scholarship; and your service to your profession, institution, and community—are relatively fluid in terms of when, where, and how you choose to address them. The reward system is often not immediate—in a tenure track system, it may take as many as 7 years, or even more, to ultimately determine whether you have been successful in achieving tenure. Student learning outcomes may not be fully apparent until several months or years have passed due to the longitudinal nature of the effect of education on a student's growth and development as a professional. Moreover, the multidimensional nature of the faculty role is rarely fully visible to those who are external to the academic environment, which can lead to misunderstandings of how faculty time is spent. When people hear that you teach a 12-hour course load each semester, they invariably wonder what you do with the remaining 28 hours of the workweek! In reality, if you are like the average faculty, you will be working at a minimum of a 55-hour workweek.

Many new faculty thrive in the academic environment, relishing the professional opportunities and challenges, autonomy, flexibility, self-direction, and relative independence that are inherent in the role, even in the face of multiple demands and expectations. Others, however, may initially find the unstructured nature of the academic environment intimidating and have difficulty focusing, organizing, and prioritizing their time, and ultimately their academic career. The purpose of this chapter is to discuss the various competencies associated with the role and identify strategies that can aid in the transition from the practice or student role to the faculty role.

WHY SEEK A FACULTY ROLE?

If you are in the process of considering a career change to a faculty position, it is worth reflecting upon why are you interested in assuming a faculty role. Some nurses are initially drawn to the educator role when they serve as a part-time clinical instructor or preceptor for students. They find that they enjoy working with students and helping them acquire the professional skills and attributes of a nurse. Others become interested in the educator role when they return to graduate school and work closely with their faculty mentor on research projects. Some are attracted to the lifestyle of the academic year, with 10-month appointments and the perceived freedom from work during the summer months that may be more compatible with family life than the rigors of shift work in the practice setting. None of these experiences or assumptions fully address the breadth and depth of the complexities associated with the faculty role. Because of the somewhat narrow view of the role that new faculty may hold, they can quickly become overwhelmed in their first year in academia as they transition from practice and assume the responsibilities associated with the faculty role. Thoroughly investigating the various aspects of the role can minimize the stress associated with transitioning into the role.

Several benefits are associated with the faculty role. First and foremost, the benefit that comes to the minds of many experienced faculty is the opportunity to creatively influence the future of the nursing profession and the quality of patient care through the education of new nurses or returning nurses who are seeking advanced degrees. For those faculty who are engaged in research, they value the opportunity to contribute to the science of nursing and nursing education through their scholarly contributions to the profession. Having the opportunity to share one's clinical and teaching expertise within the community through civic engagement projects is another rewarding benefit for many faculty. The faculty role is an entrepreneurial one in many respects as you can experience considerable freedom to conceive and implement projects that benefit students, the profession, or the community within the context of the mission of your academic institution. Additionally, many faculty have the opportunity to travel nationally and internationally to disseminate their scholarship and network with professional colleagues, providing personal enrichment to their lives.

The challenges associated with the faculty role are related to the complexity of the role and the somewhat unstructured "never feeling finished" nature of the role itself. Although some individuals enjoy the unstructured setting found in the academic environment, initially many find the relative independence of structuring your own days and weeks somewhat intimidating. You must be self-organizing and able to plan ahead to accomplish all that is expected of you in the role. Preparing to teach your courses, engaging in clinical instruction, meeting service commitments, and maintaining your clinical expertise require considerable planning and effort and frequently involve evening and weekend hours to meet all obligations. It is easy to very quickly become overcommitted if you do not strategically select which opportunities you will pursue. If you accept a position in an academic institution that expects you to have a program of research or scholarship, those expectations must also be factored into your work life.

What surprises many new faculty is that, to be a successful teacher, it is not enough to possess clinical expertise—you must also have formal preparation for the educator role to be effective. If you have not had some graduate course preparation for teaching, you can expect to engage in some significant on-the-job training. Despite the graduate preparation of faculty and long work hours, salary compensation for nursing faculty positions is often considerably less than what you can earn in practice. It will be important for you to consider all the benefits and the challenges associated with a faculty position so that you can make a truly informed decision about whether a career in academia is right for you.

> ### Think About . . .
>
> *Why are you interested in a faculty position?*
> *What benefits to the faculty role have you identified*
> *for yourself? What challenges?*

COMPETENCIES RELATED TO THE FACULTY ROLE

To help you better understand the full range of responsibilities associated with the faculty role, you need to have a thorough understanding of what the role encompasses. The National League for Nursing (NLN) developed Core Competencies of Nurse Educators (2005) to clearly articulate the many different aspects of the role. As a new faculty or as someone who is contemplating a faculty position, you will want to familiarize yourself with these competencies so that you will gain a broader understanding of the role. You can also use the core competencies to guide self-reflection of your current level of competency as an educator and identify areas in which you will want to seek out development opportunities. Exhibit 2.1 lists the NLN Core Competencies of Nurse Educators for your reference. Let's look at each of these competencies in closer detail.

Exhibit 2.1

National League for Nursing's Core Competencies of Nurse Educators (2005)

COMPETENCY 1—FACILITATE LEARNING

Nurse educators are responsible for creating an environment in classroom, laboratory, and clinical settings that facilitates student learning and the achievement of desired cognitive, affective, and psychomotor outcomes. To facilitate learning effectively, the nurse educator:

- Implements a variety of teaching strategies appropriate to learner needs, desired learner outcomes, content, and context
- Grounds teaching strategies in educational theory and evidence-based teaching practices
- Recognizes multicultural, gender, and experiential influences on teaching and learning
- Engages in self-reflection and continued learning to improve teaching practices that facilitate learning
- Uses information technologies skillfully to support the teaching-learning process
- Practices skilled oral, written, and electronic communication that reflects an awareness of self and others, along with an ability to convey ideas in a variety of contexts
- Models critical and reflective thinking
- Creates opportunities for learners to develop their critical thinking and critical reasoning skills
- Shows enthusiasm for teaching, learning, and nursing that inspires and motivates students
- Demonstrates interest in and respect for learners
- Uses personal attributes (e.g., caring, confidence, patience, integrity, and flexibility) that facilitate learning
- Develops collegial working relationships with students, faculty colleagues, and clinical agency personnel to promote positive learning environments
- Maintains the professional practice knowledge base needed to help learners prepare for contemporary nursing practice
- Serves as a role model of professional nursing

(continued)

COMPETENCY 2—FACILITATE LEARNER DEVELOPMENT AND SOCIALIZATION

Nurse educators recognize their responsibility for helping students develop as nurses and integrate the values and behaviors expected of those who fulfill that role. To facilitate learner development and socialization effectively, the nurse educator:

- Identifies individual learning styles and unique learning needs of international, adult, multicultural, educationally disadvantaged, physically challenged, at-risk, and second-degree learners
- Provides resources to diverse learners that help meet their individual learning needs
- Engages in effective advisement and counseling strategies that help learners meet their professional goals
- Creates learning environments that are focused on socialization to the role of the nurse and facilitate learners' self-reflection and personal goal setting
- Fosters the cognitive, psychomotor, and affective development of learners
- Recognizes the influence of teaching styles and interpersonal interactions on learner outcomes
- Assists learners to develop the ability to engage in thoughtful and constructive self-evaluation and peer evaluation
- Models professional behaviors for learners including, but not limited to, involvement in professional organizations, engagement in lifelong learning activities, dissemination of information through publications and presentations, and advocacy

COMPETENCY 3—USE ASSESSMENT AND EVALUATION STRATEGIES

Nurse educators use a variety of strategies to assess and evaluate student learning in classroom, laboratory, and clinical settings, as well as in all domains of learning. To use assessment and evaluation strategies effectively, the nurse educator:

- Uses extant literature to develop evidence-based assessment and evaluation practices
- Uses a variety of strategies to assess and evaluate learning in the cognitive, psychomotor, and affective domains
- Implements evidence-based assessment and evaluation strategies that are appropriate to the learner and to learning goals
- Uses assessment and evaluation data to enhance the teaching-learning process
- Provides timely, constructive, and thoughtful feedback to learners
- Demonstrates skill in the design and use of tools for assessing clinical practice

COMPETENCY 4—PARTICIPATE IN CURRICULUM DESIGN AND EVALUATION OF PROGRAM OUTCOMES

Nurse educators are responsible for formulating program outcomes and designing curricula that reflect contemporary health care trends and prepare graduates to function effectively in the health care environment. To participate effectively in curriculum design and evaluation of program outcomes, the nurse educator:

- Ensures that the curriculum reflects institutional philosophy and mission, current nursing and health care trends, and community and societal needs so as to prepare graduates for practice in a complex, dynamic, and multicultural health care environment
- Demonstrates knowledge of curriculum development including identifying program outcomes, developing competency statements, writing learning objectives, and selecting appropriate learning activities and evaluation strategies
- Bases curriculum design and implementation decisions on sound educational principles, theory, and research
- Revises the curriculum based on assessment of program outcomes, learner needs, and societal, and health care trends

(continued)

- Implements curricular revisions using appropriate change theories and strategies
- Creates and maintains community and clinical partnerships that support educational goals
- Collaborates with external constituencies throughout the process of curriculum revision
- Designs and implements program assessment models that promote continuous quality improvement of all aspects of the program

COMPETENCY 5—FUNCTION AS A CHANGE AGENT AND LEADER

Nurse educators function as change agents and leaders to create a preferred future for nursing education and nursing practice. To function effectively as a change agent and leader, the nurse educator:

- Models cultural sensitivity when advocating for change
- Integrates a long-term, innovative, and creative perspective into the nurse educator role
- Participates in interdisciplinary efforts to address health care and educational needs locally, regionally, nationally, or internationally
- Evaluates organizational effectiveness in nursing education
- Implements strategies for organizational change
- Provides leadership in the parent institution as well as in the nursing program to enhance the visibility of nursing and its contributions to the academic community
- Promotes innovative practices in educational environments
- Develops leadership skills to shape and implement change

COMPETENCY 6—PURSUE CONTINUOUS QUALITY IMPROVEMENT IN THE NURSE EDUCATOR ROLE

Nurse educators recognize that their role is multidimensional and that an ongoing commitment to develop and maintain competence in the role is essential. To pursue continuous quality improvement in the nurse educator role, the individual:

- Demonstrates a commitment to lifelong learning
- Recognizes that career enhancement needs and activities change as experience is gained in the role
- Participates in professional development opportunities that increase one's effectiveness in the role
- Balances the teaching, scholarship, and service demands inherent in the role of educator and member of an academic institution
- Uses feedback gained from self, peer, student, and administrative evaluation to improve role effectiveness
- Engages in activities that promote one's socialization to the role
- Uses knowledge of legal and ethical issues relevant to higher education and nursing education as a basis for influencing, designing, and implementing policies and procedures related to students, faculty, and the educational environment
- Mentors and supports faculty colleagues

COMPETENCY 7—ENGAGE IN SCHOLARSHIP

Nurse educators acknowledge that scholarship is an integral component of the faculty role and that teaching itself is a scholarly activity. To engage effectively in scholarship, the nurse educator:

- Draws on extant literature to design evidence-based teaching and evaluation practices
- Exhibits a spirit of inquiry about teaching and learning, student development, evaluation methods, and other aspects of the role
- Designs and implements scholarly activities in an established area of expertise
- Disseminates nursing and teaching knowledge to a variety of audiences through various means

(continued)

- Demonstrates skill in proposal writing for initiatives that include, but are not limited to, research, resource acquisition, program development, and policy development
- Demonstrates qualities of a scholar: integrity, courage, perseverance, vitality, and creativity

COMPETENCY 8—FUNCTION WITHIN THE EDUCATIONAL ENVIRONMENT

Nurse educators are knowledgeable about the educational environment within which they practice and recognize how political, institutional, social, and economic forces impact their role. To function as a good "citizen of the academy," the nurse educator:

- Uses knowledge of history and current trends and issues in higher education as a basis for making recommendations and decisions on educational issues
- Identifies how social, economic, political, and institutional forces influence higher education in general and nursing education in particular
- Develops networks, collaborations, and partnerships to enhance nursing's influence within the academic community
- Determines own professional goals within the context of academic nursing and the mission of the parent institution and nursing program
- Integrates the values of respect, collegiality, professionalism, and caring to build an organizational climate that fosters the development of students and teachers
- Incorporates the goals of the nursing program and the mission of the parent institution when proposing change or managing issues
- Assumes a leadership role in various levels of institutional governance
- Advocates for nursing and nursing education in the political arena

Facilitating Learning for Students

Teaching and facilitating learning for our students is the primary reason most nurses are attracted to the faculty role in the first place—they want to influence the professional development of nursing students. It is unquestionably the most visible aspect of being a faculty and the one for which we are most likely to be held publically accountable to others. As a novice educator, it is the teaching aspect of your role that you will concentrate on developing the most during your first year as a faculty. You will quickly discover that the competency *Facilitate Learning* (NLN, 2005) as illustrated in Exhibit 2.1 encompasses much more than developing lesson plans for classroom and clinical teaching. Demonstrating excellence in teaching requires the careful cultivation and integration of clinical knowledge and skills, professional values, teaching knowledge, and personal characteristics that facilitate the development of relationships with others. Let's explore each of these areas in detail.

Clearly it is essential that to be a successful teacher you must have the clinical knowledge base and experience associated with the areas that you are assigned to teach. As you transition into the role of faculty, however, you will be faced with two major challenges—how to maintain your clinical expertise while working predominately in an academic setting and how best to share that expertise with your students in a manner that facilitates their knowledge and skill acquisition. Remember that being a clinical expert alone is not sufficient for becoming an excellent teacher; there is an art and a science associated with the teaching decisions that you will make. In their narrative study of novice faculty, Cangelosi, Crocker, and Sorrell (2009) addressed the concerns of nurses who were clinical experts, yet found themselves in the unfamiliar role of a novice as educators. These nurses expressed feelings of fear and anxiety in assuming their new set of teaching responsibilities. You will find that you will need to set aside focused time to develop yourself as a teacher. We will discuss strategies to ensure a successful transition into the teaching role in Chapter 5.

It will also be important for you to consider what strategies you can implement in your faculty role that will help you to maintain your clinical knowledge base. If you hold certification as an advanced practice nurse, it will be necessary for you to factor in the practice time required to maintain your certification. You will want to determine if your academic institution will allow you to maintain a practice day during the week, which is most desirable, or if you will need to establish some other arrangements for clinical practice.

In your role as faculty, you will always be looked upon as a role model of professional values—not just among your students but also among the other health care professionals with whom you will come in contact. Your interactions with your students, patients and family members, faculty colleagues, and other health care professionals will be constantly observed by others. Being able to articulate and demonstrate your professional values in a manner that makes them "visible" for your students to emulate requires reflection and deliberate action on your part. This may require you to more consciously consider and "talk out loud" about your actions than you have been previously accustomed to in practice. Excellent writing and oral communication skills that you can demonstrate in various situations and settings will also need to be developed and honed.

The personal characteristics that you bring to the role and that enable you to develop collegial working relationships with others will also be very important to your success as a teacher. Warmth, trust, respect, patience, and caring are examples of personal attributes that are considered to be essential to the role (NLN, 2005). Being able to demonstrate a respect for learner diversity, a genuine interest in developing students as professionals, and enthusiasm for your role are other important attributes. One of the challenges that new faculty frequently experience when transitioning from practice is that of learning to direct, provide, and influence patient care through the inexpert eyes and hands of students—this is a distinct and invaluable skill that requires you to demonstrate flexibility, patience, and empathy and to *model* clinical reasoning instead of just "doing" it as you would in your own nursing practice.

Finally, facilitating the learning of students requires that you be knowledgeable about educational theory and use that knowledge to design student learning experiences; develop skill in using a variety of teaching strategies, including those that integrate technology; and engage in evidence-based teaching practices. Remember that education is, in and of itself, a distinct discipline. As a nurse educator, you are now being called upon to develop and maintain your expertise in two disciplines—nursing and education. It is quite possible that your academic institution will offer a variety of continuing education workshops and seminars that will assist you in the development of your teaching skills. Many academic institutions have centers devoted to teaching and learning through which you can gain invaluable consultation from expert instructional personnel and network with faculty from other disciplines—be sure to cultivate a habit of taking advantage of these resources on a regular basis, as developing and maintaining your teaching expertise will be an ongoing pursuit during your academic career.

Think About . . .

What strengths and experiences do you bring from your practice role to your educator role that you can draw upon to facilitate student learning? What do you believe you will find most challenging as you develop your teaching competencies?

Developing and Socializing Learners

Closely associated with facilitating the learning of students is the competency *Facilitate Learner Development and Socialization* (NLN, 2005). This competency addresses your role in fostering student development and socializing students to the professional values of the nursing discipline. One of the greatest joys of teaching is having the opportunity to celebrate the diversity and individuality of your students—although you may have a teaching assignment that requires you to teach the same course each semester, the unique learning needs of your students will vary significantly from semester to semester, creating a different teaching-learning environment each time. It will be your responsibility to develop means by which you can assess the learning styles of your students and thus develop learning activities that will respect the many different ways of learning that will be demonstrated by your students. Such an assessment will also help you provide the educational resources (e.g., remediation, tutoring, instructional materials, etc.) that are needed to facilitate student success in the cognitive, psychomotor, and affective domains.

One aspect of student development involves academic advising. Depending on your institution, formally engaging in student academic advising may or may not be an expectation of faculty. If it is, you will be expected to familiarize yourself with the responsibilities of the advising role so that you can provide meaningful guidance to your assigned advisees. If it is not a formal and assigned expectation, you will still find yourself in advising situations with students who may be having difficulty meeting the program's academic requirements, experiencing life challenges that are affecting their schoolwork, or seeking career guidance and mentoring. During your first year in your teaching role, make it a priority to gain an understanding of the legal and ethical considerations that will guide your interactions with students—the Americans with Disabilities Act (ADA) of 1990 (Public Law 101–336), Family Educational Rights and Privacy Act (FERPA) of 1974 Regulations (Title 34, Part 99), and Health Insurance Portability and Accountability Act (HIPAA) of 1996 Privacy Rule (Public Law 104–191) are examples of laws that have implications for what you can say and require of students in educational settings. You will also want to make it a priority to collect information about the resources that are available on campus and within your community to assist students who are experiencing personal crises, whether academic or personal in nature. Being knowledgeable of these laws and equipped with these resources will help you to develop the confidence needed to advise students and direct them to the resources best suited to meet their needs. Developing effective student relationships will be discussed further in Chapter 5.

Assessing and Evaluating Learning

A key component of your role as a faculty is learning to effectively *Use Assessment and Evaluation Strategies* (NLN, 2005) to evaluate student learning outcomes. For many novice faculty, student evaluation is one of the more difficult aspects of the role in which to develop a feeling of competence. This includes assessing and evaluating student learning outcomes in the cognitive, psychomotor, and affective domains in classroom, laboratory, and clinical settings.

Assessment and evaluation strategies are similar in nature; however, the data derived from each are used for different purposes. You engage in assessment when you gather data to determine a student's current level of knowledge or skill in a given area. The assessment data are then analyzed and used to design learning experiences that will help address any gaps in student knowledge or skill and facilitate students' achievement of desired learning outcomes. Evaluation strategies, on the other hand, are used to measure the achievement of outcomes with a judgment rendered as to whether students have successfully met the desired outcomes.

There are a number of strategies that you will learn to use to assess and evaluate student learning. Multiple choice tests, written essays, journaling, oral reports, electronically administered tests, simulated scenarios, psychomotor skill demonstrations, and observation of patient care delivery are just a few examples. As you can see, the use of each of these strategies will require of you a slightly different set of evaluative skills. Providing evaluation feedback to students also requires that you learn to be sensitive to *how* you deliver feedback to the learner. Just as you will have the opportunity to share positive feedback with students, you will also find yourself in the position of having to tell students that they did not meet the desired outcomes. The means by which you share this feedback can have a significant impact on a student's self-esteem and future career as a nurse.

As a novice educator, do not be surprised to find that you feel uncertain or uncomfortable with designing evaluation strategies by which to measure your students' accomplishments and assigning grades to your students' performance. Evaluation is an inherently subjective process even when objective methods and instruments have been carefully designed to measure clearly established learning outcomes. In the end, in addition to the evaluation measurements that have been taken, it is your professional and expert judgment as a nurse and educator that will be called upon to determine the final grade that you assign to a student's test, assignment, or clinical performance. This is especially true in the clinical setting, where you are required to evaluate the students' quality and safety of patient care and clinical decision making. We will discuss further in Chapter 5 how to address situations of poor student performance.

It is beyond the scope of this text to fully elaborate on all the issues that are associated with developing your competency in assessing and evaluating student performance. To assist you in this process during your first years as a faculty, it will be well worth your time and money to invest in the purchase of some reference books that will guide you in developing effective methods of assessment and evaluation in classroom and clinical settings. The resource section in the Appendix of this book includes some texts devoted to assessment and evaluation that you may wish to review.

You must also recognize that it is not easy to develop tests or other forms of evaluation tools. Looking at a completed test is somewhat similar to reading a published journal article—all that is apparent to readers is the final outcome, not the hours of work that went into writing and revising the article. Writing test questions looks deceptively simple—after all, how much time can it take to write 10–15 test questions on a topic in which you are an expert? However, unless you have significant experience with the process, it is not possible to fully understand the amount of time required to develop or revise an evaluation tool that will be reliable and valid. Not soliciting the feedback of your faculty peers on your newly developed test questions, for example, is a sure way to guarantee that you will produce some unreliable and invalid tests—and that you will determine this only *after* you administer the test and have results that you cannot reliably use to assign grades to your students. To minimize the likelihood of this happening, be sure to allow yourself adequate time to develop your evaluation materials, obtain peer review, and revise accordingly. This peer review step is essential—and one that you should continue even as you gain more experience as an educator. Taking the time to engage in peer review before the use of any evaluation measure will greatly minimize the amount of time that you will need to devote to the problem solving that will be required if you use an evaluation measure that has not been carefully vetted by you and others. As a summary, Exhibit 2.2 contains some strategies you can use to assist you in developing your skill in assessment and evaluation of student learning.

Exhibit 2.2

Developing Skill in Assessing and Evaluating Student Learning

- Read literature to increase knowledge of assessment and evaluation strategies
- Choose the strategy most appropriate for measuring desired learning outcomes
- Attend test construction and item-writing workshops
- Enroll in an academic or continuing education evaluation course
- Develop grading rubrics to use as a guide in the evaluation process
- Seek peer review of your evaluation strategy *prior* to using the strategy with students

---

Think About . . .

What assessment and evaluation strategies have you developed competence in as a practitioner that you can transfer to the academic setting?

Developing and Evaluating Curriculum and Program Outcomes

The first three competencies that we have discussed—facilitating student learning, facilitating student development and socialization, and assessing and evaluating student outcomes—have focused on the aspects of the faculty role that directly involve your interactions with students in the teaching-learning process. As a new faculty with limited teaching experience, you will devote considerable time in your first year to developing your skills in these three areas. However, there are other responsibilities of the faculty role that also impact student learning outcomes and, ultimately, program outcomes from a more systematic perspective. Engaging in curriculum development and program evaluation is one such faculty responsibility. As a new faculty, the degree to which you will initially be involved in curriculum development will depend on your institutional setting and the needs that exist within that environment. If you are faculty in a program that has a fairly well-established curriculum, you may not initially be asked to engage in much curriculum work beyond what is applicable to your own courses. However, if you are teaching in a program that is engaged in widespread curriculum revision, you may be expected to participate more fully in the process even as a novice educator. In academic environments, collaboratively deciding what the curriculum should consist of is considered to be the right and responsibility of faculty, so at some point you will undoubtedly be engaged in curriculum development activities. In order for the curriculum to remain relevant and responsive to the demands of contemporary practice, it must be dynamic and evaluated at regular intervals. Because of this need, faculty do devote a significant amount of time to discussing "the curriculum." This is usually accomplished through the actions of a curriculum committee.

Another expected competency of faculty is to *Participate in Curriculum Design and Evaluation of Program Outcomes* (NLN, 2005).

Curriculum design and program evaluation encompass a wide variety of activities and differing levels of expertise on the part of faculty. Some activities are at the individual course level while others are focused at the systemic program level. Regardless of the level at which the curriculum development activity occurs, a well-designed curriculum must function as an integrated whole. Therefore, any curriculum changes made at the program level have the potential to impact your courses, and any changes you make at the course level have the potential to impact other courses and ultimately program outcomes. It is your responsibility to remain fully informed of all curriculum decisions made by the collective faculty.

Examples of curriculum activities that you might find yourself engaged in as a new faculty include developing student learning outcomes, choosing learning activities, and identifying evaluation strategies for your assigned courses (NLN, 2005). As you gain further experience in curriculum development, you may also be expected to participate in more system-level curriculum work, such as writing program outcomes and competencies that are integrated throughout the curriculum to help students attain these outcomes. If you have not had any academic preparation in curriculum development, you will want to consider enrolling in a curriculum course to increase your understanding of curriculum design and program evaluation.

Evaluation of program outcomes requires the systematic collection of evaluation data, which enables faculty to make decisions about how well the program outcomes are being demonstrated by graduates of the program. As faculty, your role in this process will be to participate in collecting individual course evaluation data as requested. Typically, programs have evaluation committees or administrators who have been appointed to coordinate this work of the faculty.

As part of your responsibilities for maintaining curriculum integrity, it will be important for you to understand what curriculum elements you have the autonomy to change as an individual faculty member and what changes require the approval of the collective nursing faculty as well as campus-level approvals. Although the process may vary from institution to institution, you will most likely have the right to alter unit or module learning objectives, learning activities, and evaluation strategies. You will not have the right to change course numbers, course descriptions, or course-level objectives without the approval of the faculty or the institution. In addition, if your courses have been assigned specific topical content areas, you do not have the singular authority to eliminate those topics or refuse to teach them without due consideration by all faculty. Think of the curriculum as a road map to a destination, with the destination being the achievement of program outcomes. If the faculty located along the road make individual decisions to alter the way to the destination without communicating those decisions to the other faculty, students may not receive the learning experiences they need to arrive at the predetermined location—which is to achieve the program outcomes. Maintaining the integrity of the curriculum is the responsibility of all faculty, and as you develop further competence with curriculum development and evaluation, this part of your faculty role will grow in significance.

Think About . . .

What are some strategies that you can use to further develop your knowledge about curriculum development and program evaluation?

Becoming a Change Agent and Leader

In your role as a faculty, you will be expected to *Function as a Change Agent and Leader* (NLN, 2005). This is a competency that will develop for you over a period of time. You will be able to develop in this competency as you acclimate to the academic environment and become more familiar with the full scope of your responsibilities as a faculty. Even if you have been used to functioning as a leader and change agent in the practice environment, the academic environment has a very different culture from the practice setting, and it will take some time for you to adjust to the expectations of that environment. Being a change agent in the academic environment will require you to develop not only an understanding of issues affecting nursing education but also an understanding of academic organizational structures, faculty governance, academic change process, and higher education.

The academic environment is one that embraces diversity of opinion and, in fact, celebrates and encourages this diversity. Achieving consensus among faculty, who typically value their independence from administration, can be challenging, and the organizational dynamics created by these challenges will be reflected in the environment. To emerge as a leader among faculty takes time, and you will need to first fully understand the academic culture that you have entered. You can gain a clearer understanding of the culture by attending faculty council governance meetings within the school and at the campus level and by participating on faculty governance committees as appropriate. Ask your department chairperson, director, or dean for guidance in determining which of these activities would be most beneficial for you to attend.

Opportunities to participate in leadership and change agent activities are not limited to the academic environment, nor are they limited to formal administrative appointments. It is very common for faculty expertise to be sought out by health care agencies with requests to provide consultation around any number of issues. Faculty are also frequently sought out to serve as advocates for the profession and for health care, especially in the area of health care policy development. Nursing faculty may also be asked to serve on task forces or governing boards of professional nursing organizations, which is another means by which to influence change within the profession. These are just a few examples of the many ways you can develop your leadership and change agent skills. You can begin by seeking out local leadership opportunities in your area of expertise and, as you gain experience, gradually seek activities that are regional, national, or international in nature.

Think About . . .

How would you assess your current level of leadership and change agent skills? How might you apply those skills to your new role as a faculty?

Ongoing Development in the Nurse Educator Role

When you make the transition to the faculty role, you are making a commitment to lifelong learning. As a practitioner, you are already familiar with the need to be committed to staying current in clinical practice. In the faculty role, the areas in which you must stay current expand. You will soon discover that you are making a commitment to staying current not only in clinical practice but also in education, policy development, and health care system trends as well. To maintain competence in your role, it will be essential that you make a commitment to *Pursue Continuous Quality Improvement in the Nurse Educator Role* (NLN, 2005). Continuous quality improvement means that you acknowledge the need to continually seek out ways to improve your effectiveness in all aspects of the faculty role.

As a novice educator, you will want to initially seek out opportunities to become socialized to the role of faculty. Attending the school and campus orientation programs provided for new faculty should be a priority for you. If you have an assigned mentor, be sure to establish regular meeting times with him or her so that you can discuss your adjustment to your new role and identify professional development opportunities that are suitable for this stage of your academic career. Your immediate supervisor is also an invaluable source of information and support during the first few months in the role. Workshops and conferences offered by your institution will also be helpful to acclimating you to the role of faculty.

Performance evaluation will play a prominent role in your academic career. First of all, you will be annually evaluated by your supervisor. You can expect to have your performance reviewed in the three areas of faculty responsibility—teaching, research, and service. The emphasis that is placed on each of these areas in your annual review will be dependent on the mission of your institution and school. Use this time to discuss and establish teaching, scholarship, and service goals that will be achievable within the next year and maintain an appropriate balance among the three categories.

You will also be expected to obtain student evaluations, typically each semester, in all of the courses that you teach. Review the student comments and identify areas of strength that you can capitalize upon as you continue to develop as a teacher and areas that you will want to improve. The first few times that you review your student evaluations you may find it helpful to have a more experienced faculty review the comments along with you to help you put them into perspective, especially if you receive feedback from students that is not constructively framed. Although such feedback can be hurtful, the important "takeaway" point is to not be discouraged but to learn from the comments. A more experienced faculty can help you identify any themes in the evaluation that you will want to attend to and possibly construct a plan for further development. For promotion and tenure decisions, you can anticipate that you will be expected to summarize and share your student evaluations with the promotion and tenure review committees. You will want to organize and maintain your student evaluations as you will need to make reference to them in any applications for merit, promotion, or tenure decisions.

Another form of performance evaluation is peer evaluation of your teaching. Obtaining feedback from your peers about your teaching is another expectation in many institutions. Having your peers observe your teaching in the classroom and clinical settings is a valuable way to gain feedback on your performance. You can request a peer review from your nursing faculty colleagues or from campus peers who possess an expertise in an area that you wish to develop further in your teaching practices. As with your student evaluations, save all peer reviews so that you can share them as necessary for any merit, promotion, or tenure decisions.

And finally, self-reflection and self-evaluation are also crucial to your success in the role. Taking time to reflect on your goals and your progress toward meeting those goals will help you stay on target. Allowing time for self-reflection will also help you identify resources that you will want to seek out for further growth and development in your new role.

Think About . . .

What type of activities do you think will be most helpful in helping you socialize to your new role as a faculty?

Participating in Scholarship

In your clinical practice role, you may not have been expected to participate in scholarship to any great extent. In your new role as a nursing faculty, you will likely be expected to engage in some form of scholarship. This expectation can range anywhere from investigating new teaching practices for use in classroom or clinical settings to having a full-fledged research career in which you acquire federal funding to support your program of research. How research and scholarship will factor into your faculty role will be heavily dependent on your institutional setting.

Engaging in Scholarship has been broadly defined by the NLN (2005) to include such activities as evidence-based teaching, disseminating your knowledge about nursing and teaching to diverse audiences, developing skill in proposal writing, and exhibiting scholarly attributes as a professional. During your first year of practice as a nurse educator, you will want to gain an understanding of the expectations related to scholarship in your institution, identify your area of scholarly focus, and identify the resources that you will need to help you be successful in meeting your scholarship goals. For many new faculty, if you are able to accomplish those three goals in the first year, you will be successful. How to develop as a scholar is discussed more fully in Chapter 6.

Understanding the Academic Environment

Undoubtedly one of the most significant challenges for you during your first year of teaching will be acclimating to the academic environment and being able to *Function Within the Educational Environment* (NLN, 2005). Academic environments function much differently than do practice environments, and academic environments within themselves can vary in significant ways. It will be very important for you to gain an understanding of the internal and external forces affecting your specific educational environment so that you can learn to function most effectively within it.

Strategies that can help you acclimate to the educational environment include reading the higher education literature to gain a better understanding of the issues influencing higher education; networking across disciplines on campus to develop an understanding of faculty governance and the campus's political issues; and becoming more astute about the legislative issues being debated within your state that will influence health care, nursing, and higher education. Identifying the informal and formal leaders in your school is another important step in acclimating to your new environment.

At first glance, it may appear that it takes a "lifetime" in the academic environment to make a decision and implement it, at least as it compares to the practice environment. However, the process by which academic decisions are made is very important to the participants of the process, and you will find that most faculty will expect to engage in debate about which course of action to take, ultimately arriving at their own decisions. The influence and role that administration has in this decision-making process will appear to be very different from what you may have been accustomed to in practice. As you make your initial transition into the academic setting, spend some time observing these decision-making dynamics so that you can get a better sense of the most effective way to influence change in your new setting.

Understanding the academic environment of the institution in which you are faculty also means understanding the mission and goals of your particular parent institution and school of nursing. Academic institutions can vary significantly in their missions, and as a result, the expectations that these institutions have of their faculty will also vary significantly. To have a successful and fulfilling academic career, you will want to join the faculty of an institution whose mission and goals are in alignment with your own professional career goals. You should consider determining the "match" or "fit" between your professional goals and an academic institution's mission and goals to be your number one priority when seeking a position as a faculty.

> ### Think About . . .
>
> *Have you considered what your professional goals are for your career as a nursing faculty? If not, take some time to consider what aspects of the role hold the most meaning for you. How might those considerations shape your future career goals in academia?*

MAKING THE TRANSITION FROM PRACTICE TO ACADEMIA

As we said at the beginning of this chapter, accepting a faculty position and assuming the faculty role can be professionally transforming. We hope this brief overview of the core competencies associated with the role has provided you with some insight into the opportunities and challenges that await you in the faculty role. By carefully considering the competencies associated with the role and designing a professional development plan by which to acquire the competencies, you will be taking the first step to ensuring your success in your new role.

Danna, Schaubhut, and Jones (2010) shared perspectives from their experiences of transitioning from careers in practice to careers in academia, acknowledging the challenges they faced as well as the opportunities for professional growth they embraced in the transition. They identified the distinct differences in the two cultures that result in differing reward structures. Whereas clinical expertise is rewarded in the practice setting, one's ability to publish, write grants, and conduct research is more likely to be rewarded in academia. However, they also identified competencies beyond their clinical expertise that they had developed in practice that were transferrable to academia and thus supported their transition; such competencies included their collaborative skills in interprofessional communication, ability to engage in teamwork, financial management skills, project management skills, and outcome evaluation, to name just a few (Danna et al., 2010). They found a comprehensive orientation plan to the school and their new role as faculty to be an invaluable experience. Suplee and Gardner (2009) also emphasized the importance of an orientation program and faculty development opportunities in facilitating the transition from practice to academia.

Case Study 2.1

Angela: Transitioning From Practice to Academia

Angela has been a staff nurse for 15 years. Recently completing her master's degree in nursing and seeking new professional growth and development opportunities, Angela applies for a full-time faculty position teaching undergraduate nursing students at the local college. She is appointed to the position, in which she will be expected to teach fundamental nursing skills and the initial medical-surgical nursing course. In addition, she will have a clinical group of 10 nursing students in an acute care setting at the local hospital. This is her first teaching position.

Initially Angela believes that the transition into the faculty role will be easy for her, especially since she will be teaching students fundamental nursing concepts and basic

(continued)

nursing care. As a nurse with experience in critical care and acute medical-surgical nursing, she has great confidence in her clinical nursing skills and is eagerly anticipating her first contact with her students. The first week she is on campus she is introduced to her faculty colleagues, assigned an office, and provided a course schedule that outlines when her classes will meet. She finds she will have 50 students in her fundamentals course and another 50 students in her medical-surgical nursing course, in addition to her group of 10 clinical students. She is given a copy of her course syllabi and asked to begin planning her course materials for the semester. She will need to have them prepared within the next week as classes are scheduled to start in 2 weeks. Some of the materials will need to be posted online for students to access. Clinical experiences for her students need to be negotiated with the acute care agency. Equipment and supplies must be ordered for her fundamentals course so they are available when the course begins. In addition, she needs to anticipate planning the first test she will administer in the medical-surgical course so that she can allow adequate time for the test to be reviewed, formatted, and copied. Angela has never had responsibility for planning and preparing coursework for an entire semester for one course, much less three courses and 110 students! Where should she begin? In addition, she is expected to attend curriculum review meetings that have been scheduled in the afternoons as faculty begin preparing for an upcoming accreditation visit. As Angela sits in the curriculum meetings, she realizes that she does not have experience with developing curriculum and is not sure what her role in the discussion should be. She also finds out in the curriculum meetings that she will have an academic advising load of 20 nursing students and will need to understand the curriculum plan so as to appropriately advise the students.

As Angela returns to her office at the end of one long day during this first week in her new role, she realizes that she is feeling overwhelmed and not sure of how to prioritize her work. She is not even sure how her clinical expertise as a nurse will help her meet the current challenges she is facing in her new role. Realizing she needs the guidance of a more experienced faculty, she makes an appointment to talk with her chairperson the next morning to ask for assistance in how to best approach her new responsibilities.

Case Study 2.1 addresses the feelings of being overwhelmed as a new faculty. As you plan your transition from practice to academia, consider using the strategies listed in Exhibit 2.3 to assist you. Seeking the guidance of others and using the resources provided to help you develop in your new role will be essential keys to a successful transition to the faculty role.

Exhibit 2.3

Strategies to Aid Your Transition From Practice to Academia

- Identify previously acquired practice competencies that will assist in your transition to academia
- Develop an understanding of the differences in practice and academic cultures
- Participate in orientation and faculty development programs offered to new faculty
- Acknowledge your feelings of uncertainty as a novice in academia and accept that these feelings are normal
- Seek out mentors—formal and informal—to assist in your transition
- Actively ask questions about the academic environment and the faculty role
- Seek out assistance from experienced faculty if feeling overwhelmed
- Remember, learning to teach is a collaborative venture—use expert faculty to help you develop in the role

Opportunities for Further Reflection

1. Reflect on the NLN Core Competencies of Nurse Educators (2005). Are there competencies associated with the educator role that surprised you? Has your conceptualization of the faculty role been changed any as a result of reading this chapter?

2. Which competencies do you think will be most important for you to focus on in your first year as a novice faculty? Discuss the outcomes of your reflections with your mentor and identify faculty development activities that will facilitate your development in those priority competencies.

REFERENCES

Cangelosi, P., Crocker, S., & Sorrell, J. (2009). Expert to novice: Clinicians learning new roles as clinical nurse educators. *Nursing Education Perspectives, 30*(6), 367–371.

Danna, D., Schaubhut, R., & Jones, J. (2010). From practice to education: Perspectives from three nurse leaders. *The Journal of Continuing Education in Nursing, 41*(2), 83–87.

National League for Nursing. (2005). *Core competencies of nurse educators.* New York: Author. Retrieved from www.nln.org

Suplee, P., & Gardner, M. (2009). Fostering a smooth transition to the faculty role. *The Journal of Continuing Education in Nursing, 40*(11), 514–520.

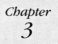

Determining Institutional Fit:
Finding the Perfect Faculty Position

Nurses in clinical practice choose to become educators for a variety of reasons. Many nurses have received the "teaching bug" when they have precepted or mentored new nurses. They find that they really like teaching and want to move into full-time teaching careers. Some nurses have had faculty members who have encouraged faculty careers. Some view teaching as a better way to combine career with family. Others realize that mentoring novice nurses through teaching is a way to stay engaged in nursing, even if these experienced nurses do not see themselves practicing bedside nursing their entire careers. Whatever the reason for engaging in a career as a nurse educator, you should engage in careful forethought before moving into a faculty position. Therefore, the purpose of this chapter is to assist you in locating a job at the academic institution that is a right fit for you. You will learn what factors to consider when searching for that perfect job and how to prepare for your job interviews.

CHOOSING YOUR INSTITUTION

The job search is an important step in your transformation to nurse educator. Many nursing faculty will be retiring in the next 5 to 10 years (American Association of Colleges of Nursing, 2005), so unlike newly minted doctorates or those with master's degrees in other fields, such as the humanities, potential nursing faculty should have little difficulty finding a position. Finding any faculty position may be the easy part, but finding the *right* position is more difficult. Although some of you may have pursued your graduate degree to stay in the faculty position you already have, others of you will be seeking your first full-time teaching position. Or, you might choose to leave your current faculty position and seek another position at a different institution that appears to have opportunities more aligned with your career goals.

One way to begin your job search is to peruse the bulletin boards in the institution where you are enrolled for your graduate program. Many universities will send faculty job postings to institutions with graduate programs. The *Chronicle of Higher Education* is a weekly newspaper targeted at workers in higher education. In addition to news articles, it has job postings in print and online. Professional organizations such as the National League for Nursing (NLN), the American Association of Colleges of Nursing (AACN), and Sigma Theta Tau International have faculty job postings on their Web sites. Although advertisements are a good place to start your job search, attending professional conferences can sometimes yield better results. Many academic institutions have booths in the exhibit halls where you can speak with those who might be in a position to hire you. Some nursing programs hold receptions at conferences. These receptions are often for recruiting faculty. In addition, conferences usually provide bulletin boards for job postings. These postings might note a way to contact a conference attendee about a position. Your faculty mentors from your graduate program are also excellent resources. They may know about upcoming positions that suit your career goals.

One of the secrets of a successful career is making sure you have a good "fit" with your chosen academic institution. Once you have decided to embark upon a faculty career, you must decide what type of institution fits your career goals. Exhibit 3.1 summarizes questions you should ask yourself. You need to decide such things as what level of teaching you desire. You will need to consider whether you want employment at a community college, a liberal arts institution, or a university.

Exhibit 3.1

Focusing the Search for Academic Positions

- Do you want a career that focuses primarily on teaching or research? Alternatively, do you want to combine both?
- What kind of research do you want to do? For example, do you want to do clinical research or research focused on the teaching-learning process?

- Is maintaining an active clinical practice important to you?
- Do you prefer to teach in a community college setting or in a baccalaureate or higher degree program?
- Do you want to teach undergraduate students, graduate students, or a combination of both?
- Are you interested in teaching beginning adult students who have had a variety of life experiences?
- Do you thrive on having young people in your office?

Different types of institutions of higher learning have different expectations for the faculty role. The Carnegie Foundation for the Advancement of Teaching has classified institutions by type since 1971. Before 2010, the foundation focused classifications not only on academic programs offered at an institution but also on the institution's focus on research based on the types and numbers of doctorates awarded. Beginning in 2010, the Carnegie Foundation for the Advancement of Teaching (2010) has a more extensive classification system that lists not only the traditional program types but also institutional size, total enrollment, setting (rural, urban, etc.), and undergraduate and graduate program profiles. The database allows one to search a particular institution or group of institutions.

Once you decide what type of institution you might like to teach in, go to the Web site of the institutions with open positions. Look at the institutional and nursing program mission statements. According to Competency 8 of the NLN Core Competencies of Nurse Educators (2005), a nurse educator has an obligation to "Determine . . . own professional goals within the context of academic nursing and the mission of the parent institution and nursing program."

How Do Teaching Goals Influence Institutional Choice?

Teaching is an important component of the faculty role no matter where your place of employment. (See Chapter 5 for a full discussion of the teaching role.) What is critical to consider is how teaching fits within your career goals. Community colleges and liberal arts colleges have strong teaching missions, as do regional state universities. If you seek employment at these types of institutions, you can expect that didactic and clinical teaching assignments will encompass the majority of your time. In fact, teaching might be valued more at these types of institutions than at major research universities. If you seek employment at a university that has a strong research mission, you may have a lighter teaching load because you will be expected to engage in a program of research.

How Do Scholarship Goals Influence Institutional Choice?

The majority of educational institutions require some form of scholarship but not necessarily interventional research. For example, regional universities with a community engagement mission might stress scholarship aimed at solving problems in the community or clinical arena. Book chapters that exemplify the scholarship of integration will be acceptable at these institutions. Program and other grant activities will also be strongly encouraged. On the other hand, nursing programs located in universities with a strong research mission are more likely to require faculty to write major grants and focus on the scholarship of discovery. At regional universities, it will be important for you to establish a state and regional reputation with your scholarship. However, at major research universities, you will be expected to develop a national and international reputation to prove your scholarly worth. (See Chapter 6 for a full discussion of the scholarship role.)

How Do Clinical Practice Goals Influence Institutional Choice?

Another consideration is the ability or the requirement to maintain an active clinical practice. Educational institutions will vary in their

---

Think About . . .

*What is my overall career goal? Do I want to continue
a program of research started in my graduate program?
What program level do I want to teach in?
Do I wish to maintain an active clinical practice?*

expectations of faculty maintaining a clinical practice. If you are a nurse practitioner, clinical specialist, or other certified advance practice nurse, you will need to consider your certification requirements with regard to the number of clinical hours needed to maintain certification and whether you will be able to achieve those hours while holding a full-time faculty position. If you are considering a faculty role and you are an advanced practice nurse, you will want to consider how clinical teaching loads and other aspects of your role might affect your ability to practice. You might also ask if the institution has a faculty practice plan. If so, you could be expected to meld your clinical practice into the plan.

APPLYING FOR THE JOB AND PREPARING FOR THE INTERVIEW

Once you decide which type of academic institution is the best fit for your professional career goals, you are ready to begin the application and interview process. Investigate whether the institution uses an online application process. In many instances, you will upload both a cover letter and curriculum vitae (CV) to a job application site on the university's Web site. In other cases, you will send hard copies of your cover letter and CV to the search committee chair or dean via the postal system. Some application instructions also ask you to submit a statement of your teaching philosophy.

Developing Your Cover Letter

When preparing your cover letter, tailor the letter to that particular job. Try to find out the name of the search committee chair or dean so that you can personalize the letter. If you do not already know the person's name, locate the name on a Web site or make a telephone call. By addressing the letter to a "real" person, rather than "Dear Sir or Madam" or "To Whom it May Concern," you are showing that you have done a little homework and are not just randomly sending out applications. Be sure to include in your cover letter how the search committee may contact you.

Exhibit 3.2 gives an example of a cover letter. Note how the applicant focuses on how her values match the university and nursing program mission statements and how her skill set is relevant to the advertised position.

Exhibit 3.2

Cover Letter

21 March 2010

Faye Grimes, RN, PhD
Chair of the Search Committee
College of Nursing,
Great Plains University
Small City, Nebraska

Dear Dr. Grimes:

I am writing to indicate my interest in the faculty position that you have posted to teach Adult Health in your baccalaureate nursing program. At a recent Midwest Nursing Research Society meeting, I met a member of your Search Committee, Dr. Sandra Professor. The information she provided me about your university's mission and student-focused environment indicates that the environment offered by your institution is one that I am interested in for my own faculty career.

I will be graduating in June, from the doctoral program in nursing education at Mid-City University. My research interests are focused on investigating factors that influence student engagement and success in the classroom setting. Before my doctoral education, I was a medical-surgical clinical nurse specialist for a large hospital system. During that time, I served as clinical faculty for a baccalaureate nursing program. Prior to that time, before the birth of my first child I was a clinical educator for the medical unit. I believe my expertise in adult health nursing and my previous teaching experience are a good match for your program needs. Enclosed please find my current curriculum vitae.

I welcome the opportunity to discuss your open position. I may be reached on my cell phone: 544.555.5555 or via e-mail at bnf123@comcast.net.

Thank you for your time and consideration.

Sincerely,
Betsy New-Faculty, RN Ph(c)

Tailor your letter to the job advertised. You should share details of the specific jobs held in the past in summary form in the cover letter when you highlight why you are applying for a particular job. In addition, state why particular qualifications that you hold make you particularly suited to the position by showing how your expertise matches the institution and program's mission statements. If certification is a desired job characteristic, highlight any certifications that you might have. If you have special clinical expertise, teaching, or research skills, also speak of these in your cover letter.

If your work history has gaps in it, you might address them in your cover letter. Likewise, if you have moved frequently, explain the moves. Gaps in your work history and frequent moves may send up "red flags" to a search committee. Search committees might without some explanation interpret these "flags" as a sign that you were frequently unhappy in your prior jobs. Case Study 3.1 illustrates how Elizabeth's cover letter, which explains her frequent moves, results in a successful job search. If you have had many job changes, how might you explain those changes in a positive way?

Case Study 3.1

Elizabeth: Experienced Faculty

Elizabeth is an experienced faculty member married to a retired member of the military. She and her family have moved numerous times during her spouse's career. Nevertheless, she was able to obtain her doctorate and was employed in nursing education, except for the time spent overseas. Even then, she was able to teach a research course in a master's program at a military base education center. The time has now come for the family to decide where to relocate. Elizabeth's job consideration and the location of aging parents will be the primary factors in choosing where to apply for jobs. Elizabeth searches job listing sites such as the *Chronicle of Higher Education* and speaks to colleagues she has met in her travels about available faculty positions. One thing she has learned from the jobs she has had is the fact

(continued)

that she wants a position at a university that values teaching. Scholarship is important to her, and she is committed to publishing. However, constantly writing and rewriting major grants is not where she wants to spend most of her time. As a result, she applies for several positions that seem to match her career vision. In her cover letter, she describes her career, emphasizing how she has capitalized on career development opportunities even though she has had to move every 3 to 4 years. Following several interviews, she and her family move to a location, closer to parents, where Elizabeth is able to develop her career.

Developing Your Curriculum Vitae

In academe, one should submit a CV rather than a resume. A CV has much more detail than a resume in terms of education, publications, research, and service activities. A CV, unlike a resume, does not list job duties, nor is a career objective noted. CVs are not limited, necessarily, to one or two pages (Career Services—Marquette University, n.d.). Your CV should have your contact information on the first page, centered at the top or in some other readable format at the beginning of the CV. Exhibit 3.3 shows a sample CV for a new graduate from a doctoral program. This sample shows just one suggested format. Your university where you received your graduate degree most likely has a career center. Staff at the center can show you other formats and assist you in editing your CV.

Think About . . .

How might I transform my current resume, which represents my accomplishments in my clinical position, to a CV that portrays my potential as an academician?

Exhibit 3.3

Sample Curriculum Vitae

Betsy New-Faculty
1333 South Street
Midwestern City, IA 502000
544.555.5555
bnf123@comcast.net

EDUCATION

DEGREES	INSTITUTION	YEAR	MAJOR AREA OF STUDY
PhD	Mid-City University	2010	Nursing Education
MSN	Southeastern University	2000	Adult Health
BSN	East Coast College	1996	Nursing
ASN	Marble Community College	1988	Nursing

EXPERIENCE

POSITION	INSTITUTION	DATE
Adjunct Faculty	Mid-City University	2006–2010
Clinical Specialist	Mid-City Hospital	2001–2006
Clinical Educator	University Hospital	1996–1998
Head Nurse	University Hospital	1993–1996
Staff Nurse	University Hospital	1990–1993
Staff Nurse	Community Hospital	1988–1990

PRESENTATIONS

New-Faculty, B. *The role of simulation in building self-confidence in baccalaureate nursing students.* Poster Presented at MNRS, Kansas City, 2010.

New-Faculty, B. (2002). *A teaching plan for sight-impaired persons with diabetes.* Poster presented at Sigma Theta Tau Research Day.

(continued)

PUBLICATIONS

New-Faculty, B. (2008). The adjunct faculty role in nursing education. *Nursing Education, 10,* 155–157.

RESEARCH

New-Faculty, B. (2010). *The role of simulation in building self-confidence in baccalaureate nursing students.* Dissertation Mid-West University.

PROFESSIONAL MEMBERSHIPS

Sigma Theta Tau 1999–Present
  Secretary, Local Chapter 2002–2004
National Association of Nurse Clinical Specialists 2000–2005
American Nurses Association 1996–Present

PROFESSIONAL SERVICE

Clinical Practice Guideline Committee, Mid-City Hospital 2002–2006
Nursing Research Committee, Chair, Mid-City Hospital 2003–2006
Education Committee, University Hospital 1996–1998
Budget Committee, University Hospital 1995–1996

COMMUNITY SERVICE

Coordinator of Senior Citizens Health Fair 2009
Volunteer at Free Clinic 2006–2009

AWARDS AND HONORS

First Place Doctoral Student Poster, MNRS 2009

Preparing for the Interview

The length of interviews for academic positions varies. Interviews at community colleges are usually 1-day events, whereas interviews at some universities may last 1.5 to 2 days. If you must travel away from your home base for an interview, you should expect that the university or college where you are applying will pay for your travel expenses up front or will reimburse you after your trip. Be sure and clarify how expenses will be paid, before you make a trip for an interview. You do not want to be caught with unexpected credit card bills!

Once you have obtained an interview, you should have a conversation with the search committee chair or human resources person regarding your schedule for the campus visit. Clarify whether you will be expected to make a research presentation and/or teach a class. If you are to make a research presentation, the custom is to present findings from your thesis, dissertation, or evidence-based practice project. You will also want to know whom will you be meeting in addition to the search committee. You will want to know if you will be meeting with the department chair or dean or another academic administrator, such as an associate dean for research. If you have special research or teaching interests, you might request to meet with faculty who hold similar interests as you do.

Another essential component of the interview day or days is a meeting with human resources to discuss benefits. If this meeting is not included in the interview schedule, you might ask about arranging a time to learn about benefits. Salary discussions are usually reserved for conversations with the dean or department chair. Before going for your interview, check online sources such as the *Chronicle of Higher Education* or the American Association of University Professors for salary charts. Both Web sites list salaries by academic rank for the majority of academic institutions in the United States. By knowing what the average salaries are at the institution where you are interviewing, you can better negotiate your own salary.

If you have strong clinical interests, you might ask to have a tour arranged of clinical facilities used by the nursing program. That way you can determine if the clinical facilities hold possibilities for practice if you so desire. If you are from out of town, the search committee may arrange a tour with a Realtor so that you may explore possible living arrangements.

Exhibit 3.4 details a schedule for a campus visit at a regional university. Note that the candidate for the position at this university not only has to give a research presentation but also must teach a part of a class. If you were this candidate, how would you prepare for these

Exhibit 3.4

Sample Job Interview Schedule

Contact: Faye Grimes Cell phone: 555.555.5555

April 21, 2010

7:00 P.M.   Arrive airport—Pickup by Faye
                             Grimes, Chair of search committee

April 22, 2010

8:30 A.M.   Pickup at hotel by Anne Smith,
                             member of search committee, and
                             travel to campus

9:00 A.M.   Coffee and meet with Search
                             Committee

10:00 A.M.   Nursing 250 Lecture—Instructor
                             contact—Carolyn Stricker—Topic
                             is perioperative pain management
                             in patients

11:15 A.M.   Meet with Gloria Strong, Department
                             Chair

12:00 NOON   Lunch—Campus Restaurant—Host:
                             Jean Miller, Associate Dean Under-
                             graduate Program

1:00 P.M.   Meet with Human Resources

1:15–2:00 P.M.   Campus Tour—Jean Miller

2:30–3:15 P.M.   Research Presentation
                             Faculty/Staff/Students—Room 416

3:30 P.M.   Meet with Dean

4:30 P.M.   Return to the hotel via Faye Grimes

6:00 P.M.   Dinner at local restaurant—Host:
                             Ruth Richardson, search committee
                             member, pick up and take to dinner
                             and return to hotel

April 23, 2010

9:00 A.M.	Picked up at hotel by Sam Davis, Realtor, for tour of town and return to College of Nursing to Beth Jones, member of search committee—Room #316
11:30 A.M.	Lunch on Campus—Host: Jean Miller
12:30 P.M.	Brief meeting with Search Committee following lunch
1:30 P.M.	Depart for Airport via Gordon Bell, member of search committee

presentations? What resources would you need the institution to provide to give your presentations?

Doing Your Homework

When preparing for your campus visit, learn as much as you can about the campus. What are the institution's and nursing program's missions, visions, and core values? Does the program or university anticipate a change in administrative leadership? If so, you might find out in an informal way if faculty anticipate a change in program mission.

Look at the institution and nursing program Web pages to determine the curriculum. The faculty profiles might tell you about the faculty scholarship interests. Some university and nursing program Web pages will contain promotion and tenure requirements. If so, examine these pages so that you have an idea beforehand what the requirements might be. The institution's Web site might also have information regarding faculty governance. A good place to locate all this information is the institution's handbook, which may be called a Faculty Handbook or University Handbook, and is usually available online.

Do not be afraid to contact people in your professional network who may be able to tell you a bit more about the place where you will interview. You might ask these persons about the work environment, how faculty interact, and program leadership. Search committees usually put their best face forward, so you may want to look a little deeper. Therefore, your informal network can be quite valuable as you pursue your job quest; make the most of it.

When preparing for an interview, you should give some thought to your dress for the day. For women, a nice suit, pantsuit, or dress is appropriate. Men should wear a suit or sport coat and tie. Comfortable footwear is necessary. Many job interview itineraries involve a walking tour of the campus. No job candidate wants to hobble along during the tour. One caveat, however: If you are interviewing at an institution that has a particular religious affiliation, you might investigate if there is a specific dress code requirement.

Traveling to the interview can be stressful, particularly if you are flying. Try to anticipate delays and plan for how you will handle travel interruptions. By anticipating how to handle travel problems, you can lessen your stress somewhat. Make sure to schedule your flight with sufficient leeway for connecting flights. In addition, have in mind back-up flights in case a flight is canceled because of weather or other issues. Be sure to have your cell phone with you and a cell phone or other number for your search committee contact. Most search committees will be understanding if your travel is delayed because of weather or other issues. If the potential hiring institution is not understanding, perhaps this isn't a place where you want to work (Evans, 2010).

THE INTERVIEW PROCESS

The interview process is an interactive process between potential employer and potential employee. Just as the prospective nursing program is trying to find out about you, you are trying to learn as much as you can about the place where you are interviewing. How do the search committee and faculty as a whole treat you? Do you feel welcome? Does the search committee leave you by yourself for long periods without any direction as to what comes next? How hospitable a program is toward a potential candidate can give you some insight into how the program treats faculty and students in general.

When you meet with your potential immediate supervisor, try to find out what your job expectations will be. What does a typical teaching workload look like for faculty? How many classroom and clinical hours will you be expected to teach? Will you be expected to teach online? If there is a tenure track, is the tenure "clock" (timeline) fixed or is there flexibility built in for family responsibilities? You should also explore what orientation program is in place for new faculty. Is there a departmental or college orientation and/or a university orientation? Will a mentor be assigned to you? If the institution is affiliated with a particular faith community, you should make sure you understand any particular behavioral expectations, such as chapel attendance or restrictions on alcohol consumption.

Exhibit 3.5 displays a list that can help you prepare for questions you might be asked in an interview process as well as questions you might want to ask. Remember, it is illegal for the search committee to ask about your family responsibilities and such things as pregnancy or other health-related issues. Moreover, if you have any kind of disability you do not have to disclose its nature because, by law, organizations must make reasonable accommodations for you to do a job that matches your qualifications. Of course, these topics may come up in conversation, but the choice is yours as the applicant to share and not the prospective employer's choice to ask.

Exhibit 3.5

Interview Questions

Questions a Search Committee Might Ask Candidate

1. Tell us a little about yourself and your nursing career.
2. What attracts you to a teaching career?
3. Have you had any teaching experience, and what was it like for you?
   a. What would your students say about you as a teacher?
   b. What do you find about teaching to be the most frustrating to you?
   c. Tell us about how you would approach a student who is struggling to meet clinical objectives.
4. Have you been on a school of nursing committee?
   a. What kind of committees do you like to serve on?
5. Tell us about your research and scholarly interests.
   a. What plans do you have for developing your scholarship?

(continued)

6. What might your colleagues say about you and your ability to work with them?
7. Where do you see yourself in your career 5 and 10 years from now?
8. What questions do you have for us?

Questions You Might Ask

1. What is your typical teaching load?
2. What types of support would be provided to assist in developing my program of research?
3. Does the school provide travel funds for attending professional meetings and making presentations?
4. What are the service expectations?
5. Is active clinical practice expected or possible?
6. In general (if the position you are applying for is on the tenure track), what are the requirements for obtaining tenure?
7. Will I have a mentor to help me become acclimated to your school?
8. Is there a new faculty orientation?
9. What do you perceive to be the current challenges facing your institution?
10. What do you consider to be the strengths of your school?
11. Depending on your family circumstances, you might ask
    a. Are there child-care facilities on campus?
    b. Is there support for spouses or partners in locating employment?
12. What are the benefits, such as health insurance, life insurance, and institutional contributions to a retirement fund?
13. Is there a faculty union? If so, what role does the union play in salary negotiations and other employment issues?
14. Are funds provided for moving expenses or equipment such as computers needed to carry out faculty duties?

When you return home from your interview, take some time to reflect on your visit. Just because you liked the people and the campus does not mean that a particular institution is right for you. The job expectations have to match your career goals. Regardless of your decision to accept a job offer, or even if no job offer is forthcoming, write a thank-you note to the search committee chair. Setting up a visit for a prospective faculty member takes a lot of time, and expressing thanks is always welcome!

One thing to note is if you do not get a particular job, the reasons may not have anything to do with you. A search committee may have reevaluated what kinds of candidates would fit best with an institution, or last-minute budget considerations could have canceled a search.

Patricia, in Case Study 3.2, exemplifies how a prospective job candidate weighs her options following job interviews. She decides what is important to her and accepts a job offer based on her career goals. Would you have considered the same things that Patricia did when deciding which job to accept? Alternatively, would you have had other concerns?

Case Study 3.2

Patricia: Changing Positions

Patricia is a new graduate from an online doctoral program. She has presented her research at several conferences. She is happy in the job she has now at a regional university but would consider moving if the right offer were to come forth. Because of her presentations, she garners several job interviews. After interviewing at one university, she knows that this is not the job for her. She values teaching; however, the search committee noted that although teaching is an important part of the university's mission statement, obtaining large research grants was the major criterion for tenure. On arriving home, Patricia writes a thank you note to the search committee chairperson and notes that she is withdrawing her name from the search because her personal career goals don't seem to match this university's faculty expectations.

Patricia interviews at another university, which is similar to her current place of employment. The interview goes well, and she discovers that others in the nursing program have similar scholarly interests and a current program grant could use her expertise. After a job offer is given, Patricia, after much thoughtful consideration, decides to accept and moves. At the new place of employment, Patricia is able to teach her area of expertise. Patricia also develops a program of scholarship that grows out of her dissertation research.

QUALITY-OF-LIFE CONSIDERATIONS

Decisions about moving to a new location are not as simple as looking at the job itself. You must also consider quality-of-life issues. Do you want to live in a large city, small city, suburb, or rural area? Will your salary match the cost of living in your prospective location? If you are single, are there social activities that match your interests? If you have children, what types of schools are important for their education? If you have a spouse or partner, will that person be accompanying you to your new location, and will that person need a job and receive job-seeking assistance? If your spouse or partner decides to stay at your old location, will either one of you be able to visit on weekends or other times without lengthy and costly travel? Finally, will you require elder care resources? Many mid-life faculty have elder care responsibilities and will need information regarding available resources in the prospective location. Not only will a tour of the area help you decide if the job location is right for you but you should also try to ask faculty questions about housing and other aspects of living in the community.

Another community characteristic you might want to consider is the availability of health care, particularly if you or anyone in your family has special health care needs. In addition, reflect on what cultural activities are available. If you thrive on things like symphonies and art museums, are these things available? Are outdoor activities such as trails and parks nearby? Do the community and campus exhibit the amount of diversity that is important to you? It is important to have accessible religious and ethnic communities with which you can identify.

INTERNATIONAL FACULTY CONSIDERATIONS

Many nurse educators outside the United States obtain graduate degrees in the United States. Those of you in this category most probably entered the United States on a Student Visa (F-1). To teach in the United States, you must have an H1B visa to obtain employment at a university or college. The process for obtaining a visa is lengthy and costly. Fees must be paid to lawyers whose expertise is in immigration law, and fees must be paid to health care providers for physical exams for you and any accompanying family members. This discussion is by no means meant to be an authoritative discussion of the visa application process but is aimed at raising a few issues to consider when obtaining faculty positions if you are a resident of a country other than the United States.

When changing your visa status, allow plenty of time. The process can take several months. Sometimes the employing institution will pay the cost of a faculty member's visa and the faculty member pays the cost of visas for any accompanying family members. Once an H1B visa is issued, you can apply for a permanent visa or "green card." The application process can take up to several years and may involve legal fees in addition to the cost of the visa itself. Be sure and plan for these expenses, which can run into thousands of dollars. A limited number of visas are issued yearly, and all involve a background check, physical examination, and interviews with consular personnel. You will also need to apply for a social security card, if you do not already have one from your student days. The university or college cannot pay you unless you have a social security number.

Visas for any accompanying family members must also be obtained. Depending on your own visa status, the type of visa the family members obtain may vary. Be sure to contact the university's human resources department for assistance with all visa matters and also view the U.S. Department of State visa home page for particulars regarding visas. One thing to note is that spouses cannot work in the United States until the faculty member has obtained a "green card."

If you are applying for a job in the United States and you are not currently a student in the United States, do make sure that you can obtain an H1B visa. Moreover, clarify whether the employing university will provide assistance with the visa application.

All nursing faculty in nursing programs must have a license to practice as a registered nurse. To obtain a license, the majority of states require that a nurse educated outside of the United States must first go through the Commission on Graduates of Foreign Nursing Schools (CGFNS). This organization performs a credentials review of secondary and nursing school education. In addition, you will be required to take a CGFNS Qualifying Exam, which predicts whether you are likely to pass the National Council of State Boards of Nursing registered nurse licensing exam (NCLEX). In addition, you may have to pass the CGFNS English proficiency exam. Once you have fulfilled all these requirements, the individual state of board of nursing will issue you a permit to take the NCLEX examination. The current cost for the CGFNS credentials review and testing is $445 (CGFNS International, 2010). Each individual state has different fees for applying to take the NCLEX examination.

Seeking employment in the United States is a complex process. Each person who wishes to teach in the United States has individual circumstances that must be taken into account. However, planning well and having patience while undergoing the lengthy visa application process can make the transition to living and teaching in the United States rewarding and worth the effort.

Nigel's case (Case Study 3.3) provides an example of a faculty member who chose to move to the United States for better career opportunities. Note, if you are a prospective faculty member who has permanent residency outside the United States, how much Nigel estimates his visa quest has cost him.

Case Study 3.3

Nigel: Moving to the United States

Nigel is a young faculty member who has taught in England for several years. He has decided to try to advance his career by teaching in the United States. He applies for several positions. One application results in an interview via Skype. Following the interview, Nigel is offered a position. He and his family move to the United States, where he further develops in his career. His one child has adjusted to school well. His spouse has made friends in the community. She wants to work outside the home but cannot do so without permanent visa status. Nigel states that the cost of obtaining a permanent visa has exceeded $10,000. The university assisted with the cost of the initial work visa, but the rest of the expenses has fallen on Nigel and his family. In addition, he has learned he must budget for trips back to England to visit family.

JOB SEARCHING—PUTTING IT ALL TOGETHER

Searching for a job can be stressful and at the same time rewarding. All job candidates want to put their best faces forward. Trying to appear happy and confident can be difficult because you know everyone is looking at you! However, remember, you would not have gotten to the interview stage if you did not have the qualifications for the potential job. You know yourself best, so be confident. When presenting your research or teaching a class, show yourself as the expert you are.

Even if you are not offered a job or you decide not to take a job, consider each interview a learning experience. Do not berate yourself if an interview does not go well. Reflect on how you can do better during the next interview.

You may accept the perfect job offer and grow and develop in your teaching career. On the other hand, what seemed like the perfect job offer may turn out to be less than desirable after a year or two on campus. Part of your dissatisfaction may be normal feelings of adjustment to the faculty role. Functioning within the academic environment is a core competency for nurse educators (see Chapter 2). To function well, you must learn the culture of your work environment (see Chapter 4). In your first few months on the job, determine if your workload matches what you expected from the interview process. If your workload doesn't match your expectations, you may be able to re-negotiate your workload so that you will be more likely to achieve your short-term and long-term goals.

Any new job requires a time for adjustment. Be patient and consider each new experience as an opportunity to grow and develop in your faculty role.

Opportunities for Further Reflection
1. What professional and personal factors will you take into consideration when deciding where to apply for an academic position?
2. Before interviewing for a possible job, what will you want to know about an institution and nursing program?
3. If you get two or more job offers, how will you decide which position to accept?

REFERENCES

American Association of Colleges of Nursing. (2005). *Faculty shortages in bacca-laureate and graduate nursing programs: Scope of the problem and strategies for expanding the supply.* Retrieved May 29, 2010, from http://www.aacn.nche.edu/Publications/pdf/05FacShortage.pdf

Carnegie Foundation for the Advancement of Teaching. (2010). *Using the classi-fications website.* Retrieved May 29, 2010, from http://classifications.carnegie-foundation.org/lookup_listings/

Career Services—Marquette University. (n.d.). *Curriculum vitae.* Retrieved May 29, 2010, from http://www.marquette.edu/csc/documents/CVHowtoWriteagoodCurriculum Vita_000.pdf

CGFNS International. (2010). *Welcome to CGFNS International.* Retrieved May 29, 2010, from http://www.cgfns.org/

Evans, D. (2010, January 5). Campus interviews in bad weather. *The Chronicle of Higher Education.* Retrieved May 29, 2010, from http://chronicle.com/blogPost/Campus-Interviews-in-Bad-We/19503/

National League for Nursing. (2005). *Core competencies of nurse educators.* Retrieved May 29, 2010, from http://www.nln.org/facultydevelopment/pdf/corecompetencies.pdf

Beginning Your Faculty Career

Beginning your career as a faculty member is an exciting time that can also be fraught with anxiety. The key to success as a new nursing faculty member is to acknowledge that your feelings are normal and then learn how to become acclimated to your new position. If you are proactive by learning what is expected of you, you will have a smooth transition from nurse to nursing faculty member. Therefore, the purpose of this chapter is to assist you in making that transition. You will learn what it means to become a faculty member and how to become acclimated to your employing institution, and you will explore how to bring balance to your busy life as a faculty member.

BECOMING A FACULTY MEMBER

Becoming a faculty member requires a change in identity from being a clinician to being an academic (Boyd & Lawley, 2009). Change involves learning a new set of responsibilities, values, and norms (Anderson, 2009). Most nurses who move from the clinician role into academe have developed a level of expertise that has garnered them much respect. Despite your current expertise as a nurse, moving into academe may bring about feelings of disorientation and confusion. Once considered clinical experts, new faculty members often feel like novices, incompetent in their new roles.

To transition from clinician to academic educator, you must understand all components of your role. Being a faculty member involves accepting the tripartite mission of teaching, scholarship, and service. One of the first things you should do is to sit down with your program chair or dean and clearly outline your institution's expectations for all three parts of this mission. Chapters 5, 6, and 7 discuss each of these mission components in depth. What follows, however, is an overview of your faculty responsibilities. You may think of it as a quick guide to "What I Need to Know" for your first year on the job.

Teaching

For most faculty, efforts associated with teaching take up the majority of their time. Your indoctrination into teaching may have already occurred when you were a graduate student or in another job prior to obtaining your graduate degree. However, each nursing program has different ways of delivering courses, so whatever your previous teaching experience, some orientation to teaching in your new institution will be necessary. Sometimes you will be assigned to a course with a well-developed syllabus and other materials, such as a test bank and assignment descriptions. If the course has an associated Web site, some of the course materials may be located there. In an ideal situation, you will be partnered with an experienced faculty member or be part of a teaching team who can mentor you. However, you may also be put into a position where you have to teach a course that had been assigned to a faculty member who has resigned at the last minute without leaving much of the materials for the course. If that happens, do not be afraid to ask for help! Not seeking help can leave you and your students feeling like you are all drowning by midterm. Your department chair and other faculty can help you look at your course syllabus and assist you in planning your course delivery. In addition, you will want to know how your course fits into the total program of studies so that you won't omit any important content.

In addition to didactic teaching, your institution may assign you clinical teaching responsibilities, especially if you are teaching in a primarily undergraduate nursing program. While you may have engaged in clinical teaching before, you will need to spend some energy getting oriented to the clinical facilities and the units on which you will teach students. For example, if the facility has computerized medical records, you will need to obtain access to the system for you and your students and become oriented to the system. Make sure you identify a person in the clinical agency who can answer the many questions that will inevitably arise as you assume your clinical teaching responsibilities. You may also wish to set up some time to work in the facility with the staff nurses so that you can become familiar with agency policies and procedures before bringing students to the clinical agency.

Teaching is more than just preparing lectures. You will need to learn how to get students actively engaged in their learning. If you have not had any nursing education courses to guide you in the development of teaching strategies, you might wish to consult a campus office that may be named something similar to "center for teaching and learning." Most academic institutions have such centers that serve as a resource for faculty. Also, consider consulting your campus librarian. Your campus librarian is a good resource for helping you locate materials for teaching and scholarship, both print and electronic resources. Librarians can also come to your classes and help students learn how to access up-to-date materials for your course-learning activities.

Several well-respected nursing education texts listed in the Resources list in the Appendix and the content in Chapter 5 can assist you in developing your teaching role. If you have not had the opportunity to take formal courses in nursing education (i.e., teaching strategies, curriculum development, etc.), you may wish to investigate the possibility of enrolling in these courses for either academic or continuing education credit. If your nursing program offers master's courses in nursing education, you may be able to get permission to audit these courses. Taking courses for credit or auditing the courses can provide you much useful information that may not have been included in a master's or doctoral program that did not have a nursing education focus.

By using a variety of resources, you can learn how to incorporate active learning strategies such as case studies and the use of personal response systems (also known as "clickers") into your classes where appropriate. Most schools now use some sort of Web-based course management system such as Blackboard or Moodle to deliver course materials to students. You will need to learn how to use these vehicles to enrich your courses. Your academic institution will provide orientation programs to help you learn the intricacies of the system used within your institution.

Teaching loads at universities may average 9 to 15 contact hours, with the rest of your time used for class preparation, scholarship, and service. You may also be required to engage in practice to maintain your clinical competence and certification. At community colleges, teaching loads may be up to more than 20 contact hours per week. Teaching loads are discussed in more detail in Chapter 5.

The university or college may also require you to maintain posted office hours per week. These posted hours may range from two to five depending on the institution. As noted above, the rest of your time will be taken up by class preparation and the other aspects of your role.

Teaching is more than just imparting knowledge to students. It also involves helping students transition from student to professional, so part of what you do through teaching and the advisement process will be helping students learn the values and norms of the profession.

Lilly—A First-Year Faculty Member in a Community College

Lilly was an experienced staff nurse. She had precepted students at both the baccalaureate and associate degree levels. In addition, she had served as a preceptor for new registered nurses. She enjoyed working with students. She said, "Students make me a better nurse. They keep me on my toes." Everyone told her that she was an excellent role model for students, including instructors at the local community college. Spurred on by these comments and her great experiences working with students and new employees, she enrolled in the local university master's program in nursing education. For her teaching practicum, she worked with one of the instructors at the community college. As a result, she interviewed for and was offered a full-time teaching position at the college. Her first semester was rocky. She had to prepare lectures, advise students (which seemed cumbersome to her), teach didactic course material 6 hours weekly, and teach clinical 12 hours a week. At the end of the day, she was far more exhausted than when she had previously worked a 12-hour shift at the hospital. She began to wonder, is teaching really for me? She met with her faculty mentor around midterm and expressed her doubts. Her mentor helped her understand that her feelings were normal and showed her some resources to help her more efficiently prepare for her classes.

Consider Lilly in Case Study 4.1 and her adjustment to teaching. She is an experienced clinician who has had a rough adjustment to academe. She did have a mentor who helped her. However, where else might Lilly have sought help? Not seeking help when needed can lead to much frustration as you move into a new position in academe. You might also consider why Lilly perceived academic work to be far more exhausting than staff nursing. What differences exist between the hospital and academic work environments that can contribute to exhaustion?

Case Study 4.2

Maria—A First-Year Faculty Member in a State University

Maria was an experienced nurse practitioner and nurse midwife. After 30 years, she decided she wanted a new challenge. She decided to transition to the faculty role. She said, "After all, I thought I was equipped to teach. I had taught medical residents and nurse practitioner students in their clinical rotations. In my mind, that was the same as didactic teaching."

Maria searched for a teaching position, but potential employers told her that she needed a doctorate. So, she enrolled in a doctoral program. Nearing the end of her program, with just her dissertation to complete, she applied for and obtained a full-time teaching position at a regional university. When asked in her interview about what challenges she might face as she moved into a faculty role, she could not really think of any specific ones. Several months later she said, "I didn't know what I didn't know!"

Fortunately, when she arrived on campus, the instructor who had previously taught her assigned course, Health Assessment, gave Maria a complete set of course materials. Although Maria felt confident in her clinical skills, she often felt overwhelmed, as she had to figure out how to teach those skills to beginning students. She noted with a wry smile, "I was naïve to think coming into this setting would be an easy transition." In addition to the actual classroom and laboratory teaching, she had to learn by happenstance such things as attendance reporting. Nevertheless, Maria was able to make time for students outside of class.

By the end of her first academic year, she began to feel more capable. Maria had many ideas about how to make the course "her own." Maria also successfully defended her dissertation. At the end of the year she told a member of the search committee, "You asked me during my interview how I thought the transition from clinician to faculty would be. At the time, I didn't realize what you really were asking me. Now I know; and by next year I hope to be where I can do all the things I need to do."

Maria in Case Study 4.2 is also a first-year faculty member. Like Lilly, she has had challenges in her adjustment to academe, but her reaction to her adjustment seems a bit different yet these differences do not appear to be related to her academic setting. Although challenged by her transition to academe, she seems not to have such a strong reaction to her duties, as did Lilly. In fact, unlike Lilly, she did not view outside-of-class contact with students as burdensome. Why might that be, and what lessons can you learn about the teaching role from these two new nurse educators?

One thing we can learn from these two novice educators is that knowing what you need to have to teach your first class is crucial for your success. Chapter 5 contains an in-depth discussion of your teaching role. However, Exhibit 4.1 contains a list of items you will need to get started in your courses. Gathering all of this information will help you as you begin to think about planning classroom and clinical experiences for your students.

Think About . . .

As a new faculty member, what do you know as a clinician that can serve you in your teaching role?

Scholarship

How scholarship is defined will vary depending upon your place of employment. Some universities highly value all forms of scholarship as defined by Boyer (1990): scholarship of teaching, scholarship of discovery, the scholarship of integration, and the scholarship of application. Some schools also emphasize the scholarship of community engagement. These forms of scholarship are discussed in more depth in Chapter 6.

In the context of adjusting to your first year as a faculty member, understanding how scholarship fits into the total scope of your job will help you adjust to the life of a faculty member. Use your first year to identify all the campus resources available to support your program of scholarship. Many institutions hold workshops about grant writing, project management, and other things you will need to know

Exhibit 4.1

Information Needed to Plan a Course

YOU WILL NEED

1. A copy of the program's curriculum plan so you know how the course you teach fits into the total program.
2. A course syllabus that lists course learning outcomes, course assignments, content outline, and policies. The syllabus is your course roadmap.
3. Course textbooks. If you need a copy of the textbooks, you or your department administrative assistant can obtain complimentary copies from the publisher's sales representative. Textbooks often come with resources such as PowerPoint slides, test questions, and other online resources that you can adapt for your course. The sales representatives can help you gain access to these resources.
4. Access to the course Web site (if appropriate to your institution) where you can upload materials needed for your courses.
5. Information on how to copy course materials.
6. Information about how to plan laboratory and clinical experiences for your students.
7. A way to communicate electronically with students in your course. Is there an e-mail list set up through your college information technology department, or must you construct your own e-mail list?
8. Are course rosters online or provided to you in hard copy?
9. The names of persons on your campus who assist faculty with developing learning materials for students. Such persons are often located in places such as the "Center for Teaching and Learning" (or similarly named).
10. How does the library place materials for students on reserve in hard copy or electronically?
11. What are the program procedures for administering tests?
12. How are excessive student course absences reported?
13. How are student grades submitted and what are the deadlines for grade reporting?

to support your research. Be sure to attend these workshops! All academic institutions have some requirements with regard to scholarship. Universities that have an expectation of heavy scholarly productivity may give you a 1- to 2-course release during your first year in order for you to have time to establish your program of scholarship. During this time, you can write grants to further develop your program of research and build collaborative relationships with other scholars on your campus and elsewhere. If you do not get course release time during your first year of teaching, do plan to write at least one article from your master's thesis or project or dissertation findings. Community colleges also have scholarship expectations, usually associated with the scholarship of teaching. For example, you may need to write grants to support program innovations or equipment acquisition. Chapter 8 will provide you more information on how to plan your career trajectory, including outlining a program of scholarship.

Service

Nurses have a heritage of giving service. In your professional life before your faculty career, you more than likely were involved in several committees at your workplace, held a leadership role in a professional organization, and were involved in one or more community organizations. When you transition to a faculty role, the tendency is to sometimes volunteer for multiple committees. After all, there is always a great need for faculty willing to assume committee responsibilities to participate in faculty governance and do the "work" of the school or campus. You will have many opportunities to develop your service role within academe. In your first year, some institutions recommend you participate in one committee within your academic program. Other institutions suggest you focus your first year solely on your teaching and scholarship.

Clinical Practice as a Part of the Service Role

You may also want or need to engage in active clinical practice. To gain or remain certified in a clinical specialty area, practice hours are usually required. Some institutions will factor practice into your load, and others will not. If you are a clinician who wishes to practice 1 day a week, make sure that you know how clinical practice fits into the formal part of your faculty load. Many nursing programs build clinical practice into faculty loads. If you do not work at such a place, you may have to evaluate whether you can maintain your practice.

The tendency is, however, to overcommit to practice and other forms of service in your first year of teaching. Slow down a bit! Learning a new role takes time and energy. As you progress in your career, you will find your service niche. Chapter 7 discusses how to establish your service niche and strategically add service commitments to your faculty portfolio.

GETTING TO KNOW YOUR PLACE OF EMPLOYMENT

Understanding your tripartite faculty role is a first step in adjusting to the academic life. You must also learn how the institution operates. When you were employed in a clinical agency, policies and procedures were important. Likewise, academic institutions have policies and procedures. Some of the most important policies have to do with faculty evaluation. Shared governance is one of the hallmarks of an academic institution. Therefore, you will need to explore how the governance system works in your academic institution.

Policies and Procedures

Knowing expectations with regard to teaching, scholarship, and service is important for your adjustment to the life of academe. Another important aspect of your adjustment is learning about institutional policies and procedures.

Academic Policies

It is critical that you have an understanding of the academic policies that exist within your institution. Academic policies are usually clearly established to set forth student and faculty responsibilities and to protect student and faculty. For example, you will need to know how to report student grades and attendance (if required). Most institutions have an online grade reporting system. If students receive federal financial aid, you may at some point in the semester be required to report excessive student absences, usually via an online mechanism. If you have athletes in your classes, the athletics department may have a system for keeping track of athletes' academic progress during the system.

Becoming familiar with your institution's academic code of conduct will prepare you for those inevitable instances of cheating. If a student plagiarizes a paper or cheats on an exam, you will need to know the procedures for handling these issues. Some institutions use a product called Turnitin® or something similar for screening student papers for plagiarism. Learn about the product your institution may use.

Incivility or inappropriate behavior in the classroom or clinical area is another issue you may have to deal with. Be sure you know how to seek consultation from your department chair, dean of students, or the student counseling center. Managing incidents of academic dishonesty and student incivility are discussed in greater detail in Chapter 5.

Where can you find out the information that is necessary for day-to-day operations? Most, if not all, institutions have student and faculty (university) handbooks, which contain policies and procedures that provide a guide for your actions. More and more of these documents are available online. You may also receive notice of grading and attendance reporting procedures, as well as university resources via e-mail newsletters or announcements. If you have gone through a new faculty orientation, these resources are often shared with you during the orientation. Of course, remembering all that information from orientation is difficult. Moreover, if you do not remember this information from orientation, an e-mail reminder message may not mean much to you. Department administrative assistants are good persons to go to for answers to many of your questions. For example, your department's administrative assistant can give you answers to such things as how to order textbooks for students.

Personnel Policies

If you have an issue regarding student or personnel policies, be sure and ask your department chair or administrative assistant. Just like in the clinical arena, you will need to know what to do if you are ill and when you may take advantage of the FMLA for a personal or family illness. Some institutions also have policies related to personal leave without pay.

You will also need to know what holidays your institution recognizes. If Labor Day is not a holiday on your campus, for example, you will need to teach your classes on that day.

Exhibit 4.2

Selected Policies and Procedures
That Guide Your Faculty Life

Institutions have many policies and procedures that guide your faculty life. The questions below represent areas of essential information that you need to know how to access to meet your obligation as faculty. Usually, written policy and procedure documents exist that will help you find answers to these questions.

1. How is academic load determined?
2. How are courses designed and who has the authority to make course changes?
3. What are the employment policies regarding such things as sick leave, personal leave without pay, the Family Medical and Leave Act (FMLA), or personal time?
4. What are the policies for local and long-distance travel?
5. What are the on-campus and clinical agency parking regulations and fees?
6. How many office hours are required?
7. What are the policies for dealing with violations of academic integrity?
8. How do students evaluate faculty?
9. How are course schedules determined?
10. Are peer and administrative evaluations of classroom teaching required?
11. How and when are faculty evaluation documents submitted?
12. Is there a standardized format for yearly faculty activity reporting?

Exhibit 4.2 shows a checklist of policies and procedures that are central to working in academe. These policies and procedures are typical for most higher education institutions. Knowing in advance how to access these policies can make your life easier should an instance arise when you need the information contained in them.

Travel and Faculty Development Policies

Faculty development funds and travel support policies are important to your development as a teacher and scholar. Many institutions have established policies that govern when you will be eligible to receive development and travel fund support. Such funds usually exist to support your travel to conferences, especially to present your scholarship.

You will need to know about what travel and reimbursement policies exist within your institution. What are the reimbursement policies for your travel to conferences or clinical sites? Some institutions require a travel authorization form to be filed for local travel to clinical agencies, as well as trips to conferences. Often an institutional human resources Web site houses these policies.

Faculty Evaluation

Aside from institutional policies that address day-to-day operations, policies regarding faculty evaluation are also important. Early on in your first semester of your faculty appointment, find out when you need to turn in a yearly portfolio of your accomplishments. Keep track of all your accomplishments from the first day you begin your new position. In Chapter 8 you will find a further discussion about how to document your accomplishments.

The due dates usually vary according to whether you are in your first, second, or third year or beyond of your academic appointment. For example, first-year documents may need to be submitted as early as October if the institution follows the American Association of University Professors (2006) guidelines for retention of faculty.

Included in your portfolio will be a statement of your accomplishments; CV; and evidence of teaching, research, and service. To show evidence of your teaching, include your syllabi, examples of assignments, and student and peer evaluations. Because the date for turning in your portfolio in the first year may occur before the end of the first semester, students will not have had an opportunity to evaluate you using the institution's formal student evaluation system. Therefore, you can use an anonymous survey on your course Web site, or another anonymous system to evaluate you preliminarily at midterm. Chapter 8 discusses in more depth about your career trajectory within the context of tenure decisions.

Some universities require all faculty to turn in an annual report of activities. Depending upon your institution's policies, you may be asked to submit this information in a hard copy format or through an online system such as Digital Measures®. Be sure you know the deadlines for submitting this information and the preferred format. Exhibit 8.1 in Chapter 8 gives a list of evidence you may be asked to include in your annual evaluation and tenure dossiers.

Faculty Governance

One of the hallmarks of higher education is shared governance. Faculty have primary authority over curriculum and advisory authority over many other aspects of the institution's governance. Each institution has its own form of faculty governance, and you will want to find out how faculty governance works in your particular institution. One means by which you can determine how faculty governance operates in your institution is to ask for a copy of the institutional and program faculty bylaws. This document typically lists all faculty governance committees, some of which will have significant importance to you in your role. For example, you should find out what committees, if any, review your yearly faculty evaluation portfolios. Members of those committees can then give you guidance on how to prepare your materials for submission.

Other important committees are departmental, college, and university curriculum committees. You will need to know what latitude you have in changing a course and what changes must be submitted to appropriate committees. For example, a change in textbooks, in some schools, is the personal choice of the course faculty. In other schools, curriculum committees choose textbooks for courses. Curriculum committees, more often than not, approve course catalog descriptions and course outcomes. Curriculum committees may also approve content maps for an entire program of study. As an example, Figure 4.1 shows a sample flowchart used within a nursing program for obtaining approval of recommended substantive curriculum changes. Similarly, if you were to have a suggestion for a curriculum change in your program, you would need to know the process for making change.

Most institutions have some overarching faculty governance committee named the faculty senate or faculty council. This group consists of representatives from the various academic units on campus and generally approves policies that affect faculty and students. The faculty senate also may approve new academic programs before the board of

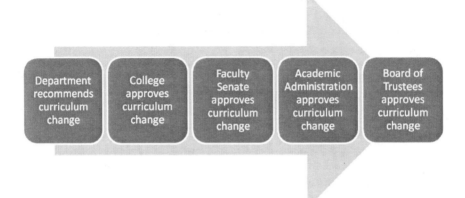

FIGURE 4.1: Example flowchart for Substantive Curriculum Approvals.

trustees or a similar body gives final approval. The board of trustees typically act only on substantive changes to academic programs, such as the addition or suspension of a program, as curriculum development is considered to be the responsibility of the faculty. Many academic programs also have their own version of a faculty council to provide governance within the program.

The board of trustees or a similar group has the overall fiduciary responsibility for an institution. In addition to approving academic programs, the board approves the institutional budget and personnel decisions such as hiring and tenure and promotion decisions.

BE A PART OF THE TEAM

Part of getting used to a new job is becoming a part of the team. Many faculty, including yourself, may have a tendency to be introverted (Boice, 2000), yet when you make an effort to interact with your colleagues, you are more apt to be viewed in a favorable light. Interaction, of course, frequently takes place in the context of formal departmental meetings. Often, new faculty are reluctant to speak up in these meetings for fear of rejection, or worse, they fear an unfavorable tenure decision or nonrenewal of contract if they were to offend their colleagues. You can, however, in a nonconfrontational way, share your own ideas about subjects in which you have some expertise or ask for clarification if you don't understand something said in meetings.

Other formal gatherings in which appearances are important include campus receptions such as the beginning of school gatherings, or open houses at the dean's or department chair's home. Although these affairs are somewhat obligatory, they do give you the opportunity to meet people and network with colleagues, getting to know them as individuals.

The informal day-to-day gatherings are also important. If the custom is for faculty to eat lunch in a lounge, occasionally join them. Gather other new faculty or your teaching team and go to lunch or for coffee. Just staying in your office all day with the door closed can create feelings of isolation, and small issues in your mind can become inadvertently large. So get out of your office and get to know others in and outside your department.

Pay attention to how the lines of communication occur within your institution so that you do not accidentally embarrass yourself. Some institutions are very structured and any questions asked must go through the chain of command. In other institutions the communication structure is less formalized, and you may even ask the president a question as he or she walks across campus.

Stay current and know what is happening on campus. Read the campus newspaper and e-mail news updates. You might find out about an activity outside your own department that interests you. By participating in those activities, you have opportunities to widen your network of potential colleagues and learn something new at a lecture or have fun at a play or concert.

BALANCING THE LOAD

First-year faculty often struggle with balancing all that is expected in the faculty role. Prior jobs in the clinical arena may have involved defined work hours. Academe is different. Our jobs can be done, in many instances, anytime, anywhere via laptops and smart phones. Being able to work in multiple venues can be helpful to you in managing your time. On the other hand, if you do not organize your time well, you can easily work 10 to 12 hours a day, 7 days a week—hardly a balanced lifestyle. We all know that is not healthy! Even in this first year of a new role, you will want to find a way to manage your work responsibilities while having time for your family, friends, and own personal interests. In an era of instant communications, many students, faculty, and administrators expect instant answers to questions. Take control of your life and decide how you will manage expectations of others and when you will find it most convenient to answer those myriad of e-mails. No one strategy works for all. Some faculty believe that they need to keep up with e-mail and course discussion boards only during designated times of the day or evening. They do not pay attention to electronic communication outside of those times. Others are more efficient doing e-mail and course activities continuously throughout the day. For example, if you have young children, you may find doing e-mail first thing in the morning at work or after putting the children to bed works best for your particular schedule. Your colleagues and students will rapidly learn when you will respond to their queries. Students, in particular, like to know in advance when and how you will communicate with them. Be sure to tell them when they can expect responses from you. During course orientation is a good time to share this information. If you will be out of touch due to travel, let the students know so that they won't complain to your department chair about your being missing in action!

Teaching activities, no doubt, will consume most of your time during your first year as a new faculty member. You must prepare class presentations and make clinical assignments. Using the resources that come with the textbooks you are using as a basis for class preparation can shorten the preparation time. However, you will want to be sure to evaluate the quality of the textbook resources before using them. As you become more comfortable in your role, you will begin to personalize your presentations. You can use your newly developed presentations in future classes, when you are updating course materials. Like elementary and secondary teachers, grading may take place at home because you may not be able to find time to grade student papers in the office.

Aside from your classes and clinical teaching, each institution has different expectations for your presence on campus. Most universities and colleges require that you post office hours and be present those times. Of course, you are expected to be present for the required departmental and other committee meetings. Aside from that, depending upon the organizational culture, you may be able to work at home at other times. If you live some distance from campus, some institutions will allow you to be on campus only 2 to 3 days a week. Such an arrangement saves on transportation costs. With the availability of broadband Internet connections, most faculty find that they can remain productive at home.

It is true, working at home can allow you to do such things as laundry while you write or prepare for classes. However, if you are one who requires structure, you may want to work only in your office, where you will not be faced with the distractions of home life. If you choose this option, or if your institution does not allow you to work at home, plan your workweek to allow for some closed-door time so that you can concentrate on the task at hand. Also, remember that working at home can distance yourself from your colleagues, and you may experience a feeling of isolation. During your first year in your new role, you may find that being physically present on campus will help you acclimate more rapidly to your new institution and the academic culture and allow you to network with others more easily.

Whatever your work style, new faculty often ask, "How do I get everything done?" Time management is key! No single time management strategy is good for all. Each of you has to develop a strategy that fits your own personality. Some advocate doing a single task and then moving on to another. Others acknowledge that some multitasking does work. Task lists work for some, and calendar reminders work for others. Most would agree, however, that you must make a concerted effort to carve out time for writing and other scholarly activities, if scholarship is an expectation. Although most community colleges do not have publication expectations, some do encourage this venture and some, as noted previously, encourage grant writing. For any task that requires significant writing time, whether it be for your own scholarly productivity or curriculum work such as writing an accreditation report, or even class preparation time, you must regularly schedule time for such activity within your workweek to get it accomplished. Otherwise, you will quickly find yourself feeling overwhelmed by the multiple demands on your time.

With teaching responsibilities taking the majority of your time, scholarship often gets relegated to last on the list of things to be accomplished. Some may find that writing every day for 10 to 15 minutes, no matter what, works best for them. Others may find that setting aside one day or part of a day, each week, for scholarly activities works better. One thing is certain: Do not let fear of failure prevent you from starting your scholarly activities. All experienced faculty have tales to share about articles rejected for publication and grants that had to be rewritten several times before funding was obtained. The most important thing you must do is start writing manuscripts and other scholarly works, such as grants and abstracts. Submit abstracts for poster and paper presentations at conferences. You can then develop accepted presentations into formal manuscripts to be submitted for publication.

Service commitments should be few for a first-year faculty member. You may wish to limit your service commitments to a committee or two within your school. Yes, you only have 24 hours in a day, and as you journey through your faculty career you may find the need to reevaluate where you will place your efforts. For example, early in your career as a faculty member at a community college, teaching will be your major focus; however, later on you may work on writing program grants. If you work at a university that has high expectations for publications, your first few years may be focused upon developing your identity as a scholar, as well as learning how to be a teacher. Remember, as discussed in Chapter 3, choosing the right job helps you to focus your career on the parts of the faculty role you value most and find most rewarding.

One way to better balance all the parts of your faculty role is to combine them whenever possible. Since teaching will take the better part of your time, reflect upon your teaching by doing some formal evaluation of a teaching innovation. Then submit the evaluation results in an abstract for a conference and then develop the conference presentation into a publication. By building on that one innovation, you are maximizing your time on task to meet multiple needs related to teaching and scholarship.

Think About . . .

How can you capitalize on your clinical teaching responsibilities as a basis for a research project?

If your institution places more value on the traditional scholarship of discovery (knowledge generation), use the clinical settings available to you to build partnerships that may lead to clinical research questions that you can develop into a grant proposal.

Personal Time

Now, you may be asking, "What personal time? I am spending day and night just trying to keep up with my assigned duties." If you can identify with this quote, you are not alone. Yes, at certain times of the semester, such as just before and during finals week, you may have to stay longer at your place of work and take more papers home to grade. Right before a term starts, you may also spend more working hours as you prepare your classes. However, in the main, you should regularly be able to plan personal time for yourself. For example, decide when it is best for you to exercise. Are you a morning person? Perhaps 30 minutes to an hour on most mornings will help you keep in shape. If you are an evening person, schedule the same amount of time during the evening hours. Perhaps you can make use of campus exercise facilities or activities during a break in your workday. On the other hand, scheduling an evening out with friends or a spouse will also allow you more energy for your work life. Pursuing special interests or hobbies that are unrelated to your work life can also be a key element to providing life balance and maintaining energy levels. Too much focus on work without scheduled periods of relaxation can quickly lead to burnout in your faculty role.

Faculty who have family care responsibilities are faced with special challenges. Research and experience tell us that women faculty members seem to have the heavier family and home responsibilities. Therefore, planning for the "out of ordinary" is the best course of action. When arranging child care, anticipate that children will become ill. Your classes and clinical sessions will still need to be taught. How will you arrange to care for a sick child? Do you have a neighbor, friend, partner, or spouse who can assist you? Can you rearrange your schedule to work at home when you have a sick child? If you have elder care responsibilities, you also need to have backup plans for care. In this case, many communities have aging centers that can assist you with needed resources for elders.

Each person has to decide how to incorporate family life into work life. No one strategy works for all. Only you can decide if you need to attend all the sports events for your children. You may be able, upon occasion, to bring a child to class with you if that child can behave appropriately in class and campus policy permits. Another strategy for incorporating family into work life is to make homework a family event. Paper grading can go on at the same time as a child is doing math homework. By combining some work and family activities, you may have more time to give your full attention to the family when needed and likewise full attention to your work when needed.

Exhibit 4.3

Schedule Example for Selected Days for a "Morning Person" Who Works at a Regional State University

Monday

5:30–6:30 A.M.	Go to gym
6:30 A.M.	Go home to shower
7:00 A.M.	Wake kids and get them ready for school
8:00 A.M.	Drop kids off at school and head to work
9:00 A.M.–12 NOON	Class
12:15–1:00 P.M.	Lunch
1:15–3:00 P.M.	Office time
3:15–5:00 P.M.	Prepare for clinical day on Tuesday
5:30 P.M.	Pick up kids at after-school child care
6:00 P.M.	Soccer practice
7:15 P.M.	Dinner and homework
8:30 P.M.	Bedtime for children
9:00 P.M.	E-mail and personal reading time

Tuesday

5:00 A.M.	Get up and shower
5:45 A.M.	Get kids up and ready for school
6:30 A.M.	Drop kids off at before-school child care
7:00 A.M.–2:00 P.M	Clinical teaching
3:00–4:30 P.M	Back on campus for department meeting
5:30 P.M.	Pick up children from child-care center
6:30 P.M.	Dinner and homework
8:30 P.M.	Bedtime for children
9:00 P.M.	E-mail and grading

Thursday

5:30–6:30 A.M.	Go to gym
6:30 A.M.	Go home to shower
7:00 A.M.	Wake kids and get them ready for school
8:00 A.M.	Drop kids off at school and head to work
9:00 A.M.–12 Noon	Office time
1:00–4:30 P.M.	Home for writing time and laundry
4:45 P.M.	Pick up children
6:30 P.M.	Dinner and homework
8:30 P.M.	Bedtime for children
9:00 P.M.	E-mail and grading

Exhibit 4.3 shows a sample of a schedule for a faculty member who is a "morning person" and has children. Consider whether this type of schedule is realistic for you. How could you adapt this schedule to fit your own circumstances? If you work at a community college or major research university, how might your schedule differ? Also, consider what is not on the schedule and how you might find time for things not formally listed.

Building a Support Network

No one person can do everything that needs to be done in any one day without some support. The same delegation skills learned as a staff nurse can be carried over to life in academe. We all need a network of people who can assist us in our daily lives and that includes our immediate family members. Children and spouses or partners can help with household duties. If needed, hire out the major cleaning. Major barriers to delegation of family and household responsibilities are guilt and the belief that we must do everything as if we were stay-at-home parents (Philipsen & Bostic, 2008). However, by delegating and accepting help, you will have more personal and family time.

Everyone needs close confidants who understand your needs as a faculty member. That person may be a colleague at another university or college, a colleague in a department other than your own, an assigned mentor, a person who has taken an interest in your work, or a close friend or family member. Use these people to help you put some perspective upon the issues you are facing as a new faculty member. Oftentimes, new faculty are reticent about asking more senior faculty for assistance. Most senior faculty are more than willing to help you with questions and concerns. In addition, more often than not, a person hired a few years before you will be an excellent resource. Reach out; do not isolate yourself. If you stay behind a closed door and do not ask questions or seek support, you may find yourself feeling lost and helpless.

Think About . . .

With whom can you share ideas or concerns about your new role? Who can assist you with daily family responsibilities?

Learning to Say "No"

New faculty often fear that if they say no to anything, their tenure or contract renewal will be jeopardized. As a result, any solicitation for membership on a committee or task force may be eagerly accepted. You receive an invitation to attend a lecture, but you have class tomorrow and need to prepare, yet you willingly accept. After awhile, all the times you have said yes turn into so many hours filled that you have no time to eat lunch, much less reflect upon your progress as a new member of the academy.

The first few years of being new to academe are exciting, nerve-racking, and growth producing—all at the same time! By not overly obligating yourself, handling the many conflicting emotions experienced by new faculty will be easier to handle. Be selective in your "yeses."

The recipe for survival is moderation and good time management along with a sense of humor. Let students see you laugh at yourself when you make a gaffe. By doing so, they learn that faculty are human beings, not cogs in a wheel. Remember, every experienced faculty member survived the first years in academe. With a few ups and downs, you will, too!

Opportunities for Further Reflection

1. How will you make room for "think time" for you to process your daily thoughts about your new role as faculty?
2. How will you keep track of your thoughts about things such as ideas for improving your teaching or how to handle a student issue? Will you have a special place to write these ideas down?

REFERENCES

American Association of University Professors. (2006). *AAUP policy documents & reports* (10th ed.). Washington, DC: Author.

Anderson, J. K. (2009). The work-role transition of expert to novice academic educator. *Journal of Nursing Education, 48*(4), 203–208.

Boice, R. (2000). *Advice for new faculty members: Nihil nimus.* Boston: Allyn and Bacon.

Boyd, P., & Lawley, L. (2009). Becoming a lecturer in nurse education: The workplace learning of clinical experts as newcomers. *Learning in Health and Social Care, 8*(4), 292–300. doi: 10.1111/j.1473-6861.2009.002

Boyer, E. L. (1990). *Scholarship reconsidered: The priorities of the professoriate.* Princeton, NJ: Carnegie Foundation for the Advancement of Teaching.

Philipsen, M. I., & Bostic, T. (2008). *Challenges of the faculty career for women.* San Francisco: Jossey-Bass.

Developing in the Role of Teacher

Teaching is the cornerstone of your career as a faculty, and for most faculty the desire to teach is what first draws them to the academic setting. As a new faculty member, it will be important for you to focus on developing your competency as a teacher, especially in the first few years that you are in the role. Remember, even if you envision yourself having an academic career that is predominantly research focused, your primary reason for having a faculty appointment is to teach and share your expertise so as to develop the next generation of nursing scholars and practitioners. Excellence in teaching and research are intertwined. As Boyer (1991) explained the relationship between teaching and research, "Inspired teaching keeps the flame of scholarship alive" (p. 11). Clearly, being competent in the teaching role is an expectation of all faculty.

The purpose of this chapter is to describe key components of the role that will help ensure that you experience a smooth transition into your teaching responsibilities. We will discuss understanding teaching load expectations, developing appropriate student relationships, setting teaching goals for your academic career, and identifying resources that can help you develop as a teacher.

DEFINING THE TEACHING ROLE IN YOUR INSTITUTION

As you accept your first faculty position, it will be important for you to have a clear understanding of what is expected of you in your teaching role. As in many other aspects of the faculty role, this will vary among institutions, based on the institution's mission and goals and overall faculty role expectations. For example, if you are accepting a faculty position in a community college, you can expect that your primary faculty responsibility will be devoted to teaching students. If you are accepting a faculty position in a research-intensive institution, however, you will find that your faculty responsibilities will be divided between the expectation that you teach as well as engage in research. The amount of time that you would be expected to devote to teaching will likely be markedly different in these two types of institutions.

Your teaching responsibilities are influenced not only by the type of institution in which you are faculty but also by the type of faculty position you accept, with the two most common types of full-time faculty appointments being the clinical track (or nontenure track) and tenure track appointments. Your responsibilities may also be influenced by the level of student whom you teach as well as the setting in which you engage with students. You will want to explore what teaching responsibilities apply to your particular faculty position during the interview process so that you have a clear understanding of what is to be expected of you. The following sections elaborate further upon teaching expectations or, as it is often called in academia, your "teaching load" and of what it may consist. Determining what your teaching assignment will consist of can become quite involved and, as you will soon see, is influenced by a number of variables.

Institutional Context

As alluded to previously, the institutional context in which you are employed will definitely influence the teaching assignment that you will be expected to carry. Institutions that have teaching as their primary mission are more likely to have higher levels of teaching loads established for faculty than do those that also expect faculty to conduct research to any great extent. This is not a reflection upon valuing one activity more than another (i.e., valuing research more than teaching); it is instead an acknowledgment that if faculty are expected to be successful in meeting the established expectations within the institution, time must be allocated to include both activities within the faculty workload. Therefore, faculty who have research expectations made of them will usually see a reduction in their teaching assignments.

Basic teaching assignments are calculated in a number of different ways. Institutions often will calculate faculty teaching assignments on the basis of the number of courses that faculty are expected to teach in a given semester or academic year. The usual "unit of measure" for making teaching assignments is the common 3-credit-hour classroom (didactic) course. In many institutions, faculty whose primary responsibility is to teach will be expected to carry 12 credit hours of courses per semester, or 24 credit hours per academic year; this would translate into the equivalent of 4 courses per semester. Faculty who also have research expectations made of them may be expected to carry 9 credit hours of courses per semester, or 18 credit hours per academic year, which would be the equivalent of 3 courses per semester. In both of these situations, summer teaching responsibilities are commonly negotiated separately from the academic year and will be dependent upon the needs of the institution.

Some institutions calculate faculty teaching load in terms of contact hours. For example, at some institutions faculty may be expected to have anywhere from 12 to 15 weekly contact hours with students. This may or may not be the same as the credit hour allocation, depending upon how contact hours are calculated by the institution.

While the teaching load numbers being cited here are fairly typical, keep in mind that these are only being used to illustrate common practices. The baseline criteria for teaching load numbers that all full-time faculty within an institution are expected to carry are almost always established at the institutional level, frequently by the board of trustees or a similar institutional governance structure. Individual academic units use these standards as guidelines for the practices adopted within the academic units. You will need to find out from your particular school what the exact expectations are, as not only do they differ among institutions, but teaching expectations can also be defined differently within academic departments in the same institution. Also, keep in mind that these numbers only reflect the actual time spent interacting with students in a defined course's class time (didactic or clinical). They do not reflect preparation time for teaching the course, evaluation time for grading papers, and providing student feedback, or office hours or additional instructional time spent with students outside normal class hours.

Institutional context is just one variable influencing your teaching assignment. In the next sections, we discuss some additional variables, which include the type of faculty appointment and instructional context and setting.

Type of Faculty Appointment

Your teaching assignment will also be influenced by the type of faculty appointment you have, as expectations can vary according to the position. The most common examples of different faculty appointments that can affect teaching assignments are the differences between nontenure track and tenure track appointments. For example, if you are appointed to a faculty position on a nontenure track (sometimes referred to as a "clinical track" for health professions faculty, implying that their teaching assignment will include expectations for clinical teaching) that is an appointment that typically has teaching as a primary responsibility. You can expect that your teaching assignment will be calculated slightly higher than your faculty colleagues who are appointed to a tenure track. Any merit rewards or salary increases that you receive will be structured primarily to reward your teaching achievements.

On the other hand, if you are appointed to a tenure track position, this is an indication that there are likely to be research and scholarship expectations of you. Your teaching assignment may be reduced as a result of those expectations. In addition, you may have a further reduction in teaching load in your first year or two of appointment to allow you time to acclimate to the environment, establish your teaching skills, as well as lay the foundation for developing your program of research. If you are successful in attracting funding that will pay for you to have some release time from your teaching assignment in order to engage more fully in research or scholarship, then your teaching assignment will also be reduced accordingly. Again, it is essential that you determine how your particular faculty appointment will affect your teaching assignment by asking questions during the interview process.

Instructional Setting and Context

Other variables that can greatly influence your teaching assignment include the setting in which you teach, the number and type of students, and the resources available to assist you in your teaching role. We will discuss each of these in more detail.

Setting

You may be assigned to teach a course in a classroom (didactic), clinical, or laboratory setting. Each one of these settings may have a differently assigned teaching workload credit. For example, it is typical for the time spent in the classroom to be calculated on a 1:1 ratio, with a 3-credit-hour course being assigned 3 credit hours in the teaching load calculation.

Clinical and laboratory courses are often calculated using a slightly different ratio. A clinical or laboratory course, which frequently requires more contact time with students, may be allotted more time in the teaching load ratio than a classroom teaching assignment in recognition of the extra time spent instructing students. For example, it is common for schools of nursing to require more clock hour contact time with students in clinical courses for each credit hour, so the ratio of credit to contact hours will reflect this difference. A common ratio for a clinical course may be 1:3 with 1 credit hour in a clinical course being the equivalent of 3 contact hours with students (instead of the 1:1 ratio used in didactic courses). Thus a clinical course with 3 credit hours will require 9 contact hours per week between the faculty and student in the clinical or laboratory setting. Instead of receiving a 1:1 workload credit for this course, you may receive one-half of that credit, or the equivalent of 4.5 teaching load credits.

To illustrate this point further, let's say that for your fall semester teaching assignment you have been asked to teach one 3-credit-hour course (for which you receive 3-hour teaching load credit), and two 3 credit hour clinical sections for which you will receive 4.5 teaching load credit for each section due to the 1:3 clinical contact hour ratio used at your school. Your teaching assignment is calculated to be a total of 12 teaching load credit hours, which is considered to be a "full semester teaching load" in your institution. The actual course credit hours that you are teaching, however, is 9 credit hours. We hope this illustration gives you some idea of how teaching workloads can be constructed. Having some knowledge of this process will help you to frame your questions about teaching expectations for your particular institution.

You will also want to request a copy of any faculty workload document, as the teaching expectations are usually spelled out in such a document. If you have accepted an appointment in an institution in which faculty are represented by a collective bargaining unit, the teaching load expectations for your faculty position will be definitively addressed in your contract. Be sure to thoroughly read any contract materials given to you so that you will fully understand your rights and responsibilities.

Number and Type of Students
The number of students that you have in a given course section may also affect your teaching assignments. If so, you may be assigned

a greater workload credit for teaching large class sizes. Some institutions will place enrollment limits on courses that are known to be "intensive" in student contact, such as intensive writing courses or distance education courses, or there may be a differentiation between the number of maximum enrollments set for undergraduate and graduate courses, with graduate-level courses having lower maximum enrollment numbers. Online courses may be assigned a greater workload credit, especially when they are newly developed and being taught for the first time. Clinical nursing courses frequently have student–faculty ratios that must be maintained as mandated by state boards of nursing and nationally established professional standards. These different variations of class sizes, use of technology, intensity of course expectations, and the level of student may all be considered when your teaching assignment is made.

Available Resources

The resources that are made available to you to help you teach your courses will also affect your teaching assignment. For example, it is a common practice in schools of nursing to engage in "team teaching" whereby two or more faculty share responsibility for teaching a course. This arrangement allows faculty the opportunity to share their expertise in the course and teach the content they are most familiar with, thus relieving some of the burden associated with teaching nursing courses that cover a large number of clinical concepts. In team teaching arrangements, the teaching workload associated with the course is shared among the faculty assigned to teach it.

Other resources may include staff support such as instructional designers, webmasters, and multimedia specialists who may be made available to assist you in delivering courses via technology. Be sure to use the expertise of the educational specialists around you to help you be most successful in carrying out your teaching responsibilities and to lessen the intensity of the workload. You may also be assigned clerical support to assist you in the preparation of your teaching materials. Teaching assistants or graduate assistants may be assigned to you to assist you with your teaching responsibilities. Developing an understanding of all the teaching resources that are available to you in your environment will help you to use your time most appropriately.

Think About . . .

How has this discussion helped you understand how your teaching role is defined in your particular institution? Are there additional questions that you need to ask so that you can gain even more clarity about teaching role expectations in your institution?

DEFINING THE STUDENT–FACULTY RELATIONSHIP

Inherent to being successful as a teacher is your ability to develop effective and appropriate relationships with your students. As you likely noted in Chapter 2 when we discussed the National League for Nursing Core Competencies of Nurse Educators (2005), it is an expectation that nurse educators be able to develop collegial and mutually respectful relationships with diverse groups of students in order to be competent in their role.

For many novice faculty, student–faculty interactions can be a very stressful and challenging aspect of the role. In fact, faculty who experience difficult and unsatisfying student relationships in their initial teaching experiences frequently become disillusioned and leave the role (Boice, 2000). How should you respond when a student is disrespectful to you or their peers in the classroom? What are the steps to take when you suspect a student is engaging in academic misconduct? How do you convey the news to a student that he or she is failing a course? What if you suspect a student has a substance abuse issue that is affecting his or her academic performance? In addition, how are you to respond to the parents of one of your students who repeatedly try to contact you to get a progress report on their child's academic performance? None of these situations are unique; indeed, they are commonplace in the academic environment. However, each of these situations are unique to you each time you experience them, because they concern unique and diverse students who present in your classroom with very different learning needs and personal issues. Learning how to successfully cope with such situations and how to, in general, effectively interact with students are important satisfiers in the faculty role. If you do not enjoy positive relationships with your students, you will find yourself not being fulfilled in the role.

There are many aspects to student–faculty interactions that you will need to consider in your teaching role. First, the very nature of student–faculty relationships must be understood. There are legal and ethical implications that you will need to carefully consider as well that provide guidelines for what you can and cannot say to your students. If you are responsible for academic advising, that will add another dimension to your teaching role. And finally there will be situations in which you will need to have difficult conversations with students, especially in circumstances in which the student is in danger of not progressing academically due to failure to meet course objectives or in situations in which you suspect academic dishonesty. We discuss each of these issues in more detail in the following sections.

Establishing Student–Faculty Relationships

When you are new to the role of teacher, it is normal to wonder about how to best establish positive teaching–learning relationships with your students and to even feel nervous about this aspect of your faculty role. Interacting with your students may or may not come easily to you, depending upon how comfortable you are with public speaking and communicating with large numbers of individuals whom you do not know personally. You will also need to be comfortable with establishing expectations for your students and communicating those expectations with clarity and confidence. Additionally, you will almost certainly interact with some students who will appear to be determined to challenge your authority as a faculty and question you about your expectations. How you manage such situations will set the tone for how students will perceive you in your role. What are the "best practices" that you can engage in with your students that will help ensure a good teaching-learning environment for all? Case Study 5.1 describes a fairly typical classroom environment on the first day of classes and a novice faculty's feelings of uncertainty of how to best engage her class of students. How she chooses to do so will likely influence her relationships with her students for the remainder of the semester.

A first step in establishing your student relationships is to decide how you wish to be addressed by your students and to communicate this to them the first time you meet with them. Most of the time this is a matter of personal preference, but if in doubt, do check with

Lorraine: Establishing Meaningful Student Relationships

Lorraine, recently hired as a new faculty to teach undergraduate nursing students at a community college, is preparing to teach her first nursing course. This course is a fundamental nursing course, which has an enrollment of 60 students and meets for 3 hours every Monday morning. Lorraine has been a nurse for 10 years and considers herself fairly knowledgeable about teaching principles due to her years of teaching self-care to her patients and their families. However, as she prepares for the first day of classes, she realizes that she has never had to engage the interest of 60 learners (who are essentially strangers to her) for a 3-hour time period, much less for a full semester. As the day for classes to begin grows nearer, Lorraine becomes increasingly nervous. She works hard to prepare her first lesson plan, and armed with copies of the course syllabi, the course Web site URL, and course material handouts for the first day of class, she enters the classroom. There she is met with 60 students who exhibit various stages of interest in what she has to say. Lorraine quickly scans the classroom. There are a few students in the first row with notebooks out and ready to take notes, who greet her as she walks into the classroom. Others sit patiently at their desk waiting for class to begin. There are several students sitting in the back of the room who are engaged in their own conversations and only reluctantly turn their attention toward her as she begins to speak. A number of students are on their cell phones obviously engaged in texting friends; they show no signs of turning them off even as class begins. There is one student sitting off to the side of the classroom with a scowl on her face not engaging with any of the other students and barely glancing in the direction of Lorraine. Lorraine begins the class by welcoming the students to the course, distributing the course syllabi, and introducing herself. As she is talking, a student suddenly

(continued)

enters the classroom (10 minutes late) and disruptively finds his way to a seat at the back of the room. He offers no apology, and indeed, seems to enjoy the attention he receives because of his late arrival. Lorraine continues with the review of the course syllabus and explains the course assignments that will be expected over the length of the semester. As the students look back at her, in some cases blankly with no sign of understanding what she is saying, she becomes increasingly uncertain about how to proceed. Although some students are clearly paying attention to her, others seem bored and are still texting on their cell phones, and a few even seem to be growing a little anxious as she explains the course expectations. Lorraine thinks to herself, "I know it is important that I find a way to connect to my students, but I thought they would all be interested in what I am saying. What can I do to engage them in the course?"

the protocol that is in use in your particular school. If you wish to be called Dr., Ms., Mr. or Mrs., or Professor, be sure to tell your students—it is your prerogative to state your preference and to expect your students to respect it. Likewise, if you prefer to be addressed by your first name, state that as well. The authors of this book have always invited their students to either address them as Dr. or by first name—the students can choose whichever format they find most comfortable. You will find some students will always be more comfortable using the formal salutation. Of course, you should always ask your students' preference with how they wish to be addressed as well when you are speaking with them.

Another initial step is to provide your students with contact information if they should need to speak with you outside of class or clinical times and under what circumstances would you expect that they contact you. Such contact information should contain your office number, office hours, office phone number, work e-mail address, and if you prefer, also your home or cell phone number. Providing your home or cell phone number is a matter of personal preference; if you choose to do so, you may wish to establish timeframe boundaries around which you will accept calls from students after work hours. You will also want to give your students some guidelines by which they can expect to hear back from you; for example, you may decide to tell students to allow you 24 to 48 hours to respond to all phone or e-mail messages.

An appropriate and effective student–faculty relationship is one in which personal boundaries are established and mutual respect is demonstrated by all parties. Although some personal sharing is acceptable and even to be expected when you interact with students over a prolonged period of time, it is important to keep in mind that the nature of the student–faculty relationship is one that exists for the purposes of providing a learning environment that will enable your students to achieve their academic goals. The classroom or clinical setting is not the place to share detailed information about your own personal life.

On the other hand, students may share details with you about personal life situations that are affecting their ability to be successful academically. These situations may include personal illness; difficult family situations affecting spouses, parents, or children; marital issues; financial concerns; mental health or substance abuse concerns; or even domestic violence situations in which they may be involved, to name just a few. An appropriate response from you as faculty is to listen to their concerns and, if necessary, assist them in locating campus or community resources that can help them address the situation. It is not your responsibility as faculty to become personally involved in the student's situation and assume the role of counselor or confidante. Even if you have the professional expertise to be of assistance, keep in mind the primary reason for your relationship with students is to teach them. You can be caring and supportive while still maintaining the professional relationship that you are expected to have to hold the student accountable for the academic expectations that have been established. Sometimes it is appropriate to provide students with extended deadlines for assignments or incomplete grades for courses due to extenuating circumstances; other times it would be most appropriate to advise them to withdraw from the course and maybe even the program, returning when they have addressed the concerns that are creating academic difficulties for them. Ultimately, you must remember that it is the student's responsibility to address the problem and find a solution to it, not yours. When faced with such situations, it is a good idea to seek the advice of your chairperson or other more experienced faculty so that they can help guide you in your decision making.

Understanding the Legal and Ethical Implications of Student–Faculty Relationships

As a faculty it is important for you to understand that your interactions with students have legal and ethical implications associated with them. For example, there are several federal laws that govern faculty and staff interactions with students. Three of the most prominent laws that influence what you can say to or about students are the Americans with Disabilities Act (ADA) of 1990 (Public Law 101-336); Family Educational Rights and Privacy Act of 1974 (FERPA) Regulations (Title 34, Part 99); and Health Insurance Portability and Accountability Act of 1996 (HIPAA) Privacy Rule (Public Law 104-191). We start our discussion of these laws with a discussion of FERPA, which governs what information you can divulge about students and to whom.

FERPA

The FERPA was passed to guarantee students' right to privacy in educational matters after they reach the age of 18. How this affects you in your role as a teacher is that by federal law you are not allowed to disclose any information regarding a student's academic performance to anyone, including their parents, without the student's expressed consent. Many parents do not understand this protection of their children's rights, and assume (wrongly) that if they are paying the tuition bills, they have a right to know how their child is performing. Clearly stated, before you can share *any* academic information about a student with *anyone* outside the educational institution, you must get the permission of the student. This includes not only parents, but siblings, spouses, friends, and employers as well. Within the academic setting, you may share the student's academic information as long as the information is shared within the context of an educational "need to know" situation (i.e., scholarship awards, admission decisions, financial aid, academic counseling, remediation, etc.).

ADA

The ADA protects the rights of individuals, including students, who have some form of documented disability. This may be a disability related to a physical, mental, or cognitive impairment. Learning disabilities are covered under the ADA. Essentially what the ADA law states is that it is not legal to discriminate against an individual on the basis of a disability in either an employment or educational setting.

In the case of schools of nursing, students with disabilities have the right to be admitted to a nursing program and the right to prove that they can demonstrate the required course outcomes with or without accommodations. Furthermore, students are not legally required to report their disability to the school as part of the admission process. Most educational institutions have a centralized office with the responsibility for providing ADA resources related to students and faculty, evaluating students with documented disabilities, and establishing the accommodations that are required. As a new faculty you will want to become familiar with the services that the office provides at your particular institution, as the specialists who work in that office will be a valuable source of information for you.

Legally there are a number of implications for you as a teacher when you have a student with a disability in your classroom or clinical courses. First, it is important for you to understand that it is the student's responsibility to inform you when the course begins of the need for special accommodations. If the student does not make this known to you, you are not legally bound to inquire about providing accommodations, nor are you required to retroactively alter learning assignments or grades if the student chooses to divulge the need for accommodations after she or he has already been evaluated on an assignment. Many schools have a standard statement placed on the course syllabi informing students it is their responsibility to declare if accommodations are required and where to go on campus for assistance. You will want to check if such a statement is a requirement in your school, and if so follow the recommended procedure for your courses as well.

When you are informed by a student that he or she has a disability and requires special accommodations, you should ask the student for the documented (written) evidence of the special accommodations that you are required to provide. The student should be able to provide this formal letter, which is provided by your institution's student disability office. Usually special accommodations take the form of requirements such as providing an extended length of time for testing, note-taking assistance, testing in isolation, or allowing the audiotaping of lectures. Depending upon the student's type of physical disability, special adaptive equipment may be required by nursing students to aid them in the performance of psychomotor skills. If the student cannot provide such written documentation, you can request that he or she go to your institution's student disability office to obtain assistance with acquiring such documentation.

If the student provides you with the written documentation of special accommodations, remember that, by law, you *must* provide the student with those accommodations. In addition, students are *not* required to divulge the nature of the disability unless they choose to do so. In addition, you are *not* allowed to ask the student to divulge the nature of the disability. This is considered to be confidential information that is kept on file in the university office that assists students with disabilities. You will be notified by the office that such medical documentation has been received and that the student is in compliance with legal requirements to provide such documentation to the university, but it remains the responsibility and right of the student to decide whether he or she wishes to share this information with faculty. Many students choose not to share this information to avoid the possibility of engendering faculty bias or discrimination against them.

The ADA has further implications for you as well. Even though a student may tell you special accommodations are required for your course, this is confidential information and you may not share that information with other faculty or staff, without the permission of the student. Always remember that the student has the full right and responsibility for choosing when and where to disclose the need for special accommodations. Students may not want to declare the need for accommodations in all of their courses. If you were to disclose the information without their knowledge or consent, that would be a violation of their rights.

Think About . . .

How would you respond to a student who is visually or hearing impaired who has been admitted to your nursing program? Do you think it is feasible for students with such impairments to consider becoming a nurse? What would be your legal responsibilities to the student?

HIPAA

The HIPAA, which protects patient rights to confidentiality, does have implications for student medical information and records as well. Any medical information that the student chooses to share with faculty is considered to be confidential information. As with disabilities, the faculty do not have the right to share this information with others; it is the student's responsibility to do so. Any written medical records that the school has in its possession must be retained in a secured and restricted-access location with only those school personnel who have reason to access the records to perform their job duties having access. Student medical records are not to be intermingled with student academic records. If a student undergoes a medical procedure requiring time away from coursework, the student usually is expected to provide a physician notice of the need for a medical leave and a release to return to classes when recovered, but is not required to divulge the nature of the medical problem. It remains the student's right and responsibility to share as much information as they desire, and those to whom they do share the information must keep it confidential.

Student Academic Advising

In some educational settings, faculty are responsible for student academic advising. If this is the case in your institution, you will want to initiate steps to orient yourself to this unique set of responsibilities. Serving as an academic advisor provides you with the opportunity to become familiar with the needs of the students who have been assigned to you; over the course of the student's time within the university it can be a source of professional joy to watch them develop as nursing professionals.

If you are assigned to advise undergraduate students, you will likely be involved in helping them plan a course of study that will meet the program requirements, assisting them with selecting electives that complement their major, supporting them in the pursuit of scholarships and grant opportunities, advising them about progression issues if their academic performance is not meeting expectations, and serving as a resource as they seek guidance for personal issues that are affecting them. If you are assigned to advise graduate students, your advising responsibilities will be similar. Additionally, though, you may be expected to provide the student with guidance in developing a research project, presentations, or manuscripts.

You will find that developing a process that allows you to maintain organization of your student advising records and files will help you to best meet your advisees' needs and use your time most effectively when performing this aspect of your teaching responsibilities. Keep written notes of all advising sessions that you hold with students so that you have documentation of the advice that you have provided—students may choose not to follow your advice and the written documentation of what they were advised to do may become useful! It will be well worth your time to find out who among the faculty have the reputation for being excellent at student advising in order to seek them out and ask them to mentor you in your advising duties as you orient to them. With time, you will become knowledgeable about the curriculum and program policies and will develop confidence in the advising role.

Students With Academic Difficulties

One of the greatest challenges that you will face as a teacher is working with students who encounter academic difficulties in your courses. For many new teachers, their first inclination is to question how they, themselves, have contributed to the students' difficulties. Are they at fault as the teacher for their students' failures? This notion can be further fostered by students who do not want to accept responsibility for their own academic difficulties and who *do* blame the faculty for their failures. It is important for you to keep things in perspective—it truly is unusual for you, as the teacher, to be the sole cause of your students' academic inadequacies. If you are genuinely engaged in developing yourself as a competent teacher, using the guidance of mentors and other experienced faculty as you design learning experiences and develop student evaluation measures, and using feedback that you receive from students, peers, and administrators to improve your performance as a teacher, then you can have some measure of confidence that you are performing as you should in your teaching role. There are many reasons for students' lack of success in their academic course work, and faculty competence is just one factor to consider.

As a new faculty, it will be important for you to seek the advice and counsel of your supervisor and other seasoned faculty when you first seek to assist students who are having academic difficulty. They will be able to help you consider the many factors that may be impacting student performance and leading to academic failure, and help you identify resources that may be helpful to the student. They will also be able to help you to thoroughly understand school policies that affect student academic progression in the program, so that you can in turn, accurately inform students about the policies. When confronted with these difficult academic situations don't hesitate to seek the expertise of others to guide you in your interactions with students who are in danger of failing.

It is natural that you will want all of your students to be successful in achieving their goal of becoming a nurse. Nursing school is competitive and students who have been admitted to the program have already demonstrated they have the academic qualifications to be successful in the program. But having the academic capacity to do the work required in nursing school is only one part of what it takes to be successful in nursing school. Students must also have the aptitude and desire to be a nurse and care for people. This is not always apparent to students until they get into the program and find that being a nurse (or pursuing graduate nursing education) is not a good fit for them professionally or personally. Additionally, many students have personal life situations that influence their ability to concentrate on their studies to the extent that they need to for them to be successful. Simply put, it is not realistic to expect that all of your students will progress in the program and it is inevitable that you will need to counsel students who are performing poorly.

When you have identified concerns about a student's performance, it is best that you discuss your concerns with the student when first identified, so that the student can be afforded as much assistance and time as possible to improve his or her performance. Any discussions about student performance should be directly connected to the expected course outcomes and confined to observed behaviors that indicate the student is not meeting the outcomes. These behaviors may be cognitive, psychomotor, or affective. Avoid making assumptions or speculations about behaviors or getting involved in the student's personal issues. The student must accept responsibility for addressing his or her own personal situation. You are responsible for documenting the student's ability to demonstrate success in meeting the course objectives.

You will want to share with the student the observations you have made about his or her performance, discuss with the student potential factors that may be impacting the student's ability to be successful, and work with the student to identify resources that the student can access to help address the concerns. Document your discussions with the student for your own benefit and records. You may wish to establish a learning contract with the student that identifies the expectations that you have for the student and the behaviors that the student will need to exhibit to successfully pass the course. You may also want to meet at regular intervals with the student to discuss progress in meeting the expectations. By taking these steps you will be maintaining communication with the student throughout the course as he or she works to improve performance; if the student does end up failing the course, you will know that you provided the student with a supportive environment in which every opportunity was given to be successful.

Student Incivility and Academic Dishonesty

Incidents of student incivility and academic dishonesty appear to be on the increase in educational environments. Unfortunately, you will probably be exposed to both early in your teaching career. How you respond to such incidents can have a significant impact on the outcomes associated with the events, so it is a good idea to give some preliminary thought to how you will address either incident should it occur in your interactions with students. It has also been reported that experiencing student incivility and academic dishonesty can have negative effects on faculty morale, self-esteem and confidence (Kolanko, Clark, Heinrich, Serembus, & Sifford, 2006; Luparell, 2007).

As part of your orientation to your teaching role you should familiarize yourself with the institution's policy and procedures related to student misconduct. Most institutions have adopted student bill of rights and student code of honor (conduct) statements that are publicly disseminated in school bulletins and on Web sites. All students are expected to be familiar with the documents and as faculty you should familiarize yourself with the documents as well. Both incivility and academic dishonesty are considered to be violations of student code of conduct and depending upon the extent of the infraction can result in disciplinary action being taken against the student, up to and including dismissal from the program and the university.

What can you do to lessen the likelihood of either occurring in your classroom or clinical courses? First, check out the policy related to student conduct that is in effect for your program. It is quite possible that language has been written that is to be inserted in all course syllabi addressing the possible sanctions associated with either student incivility or academic dishonesty. If this is the case be sure the statements are included in your syllabi and take some time during the first day of class to discuss the policy and its implications for students. Be clear in your communication of your expectations of students regarding their behavior and invite some mutual exchange of dialogue about "rules of engagement" for the course by which everyone agrees to abide by. Having such conversations at the beginning of the course does set a level of expectation and will make it easier to hold students accountable for their actions.

Second, civility starts with you as the faculty role model. Boice (2000) stated that incivility in the classroom frequently starts with faculty incivility, even when it is unintentional. Clark and Springer (2010) conducted a study of academic leaders in which acts of faculty incivility toward students were identified; these included making rude and demeaning comments to students and having unreasonable expectations. Always treat your students with respect, regardless of the situation, even when they may not be demonstrating respect toward you. Comments or questions that challenge statements that you have made in class are not necessarily considered to be demonstrations of incivility. Those are situations that you will need to manage with an open, patient, and calm manner. If a student does act in an uncivil manner toward you or peers, calmly remind the student that such behavior is not acceptable and that you will be willing to discuss the student's concerns once acceptable behavior is demonstrated by the student. If the student's behavior becomes threatening in any manner toward you or others, do not hesitate to call campus security to assist in the situation.

As faculty you have the responsibility to maintain a classroom environment that is nonthreatening and conducive to learning for all. To allow a student or student(s) to alter that environment is not upholding that responsibility. To learn more about how to maintain a civil classroom that respects the rights of all, be alert for workshops and conferences sponsored by your institution and professional organizations that address the topic of campus incivility. Books and journal articles that provide tips on how to manage the learning environment can also be helpful. The campus offices that address student issues (e.g., dean of students, student advocate services, etc.) are also good sources of information about how to establish and manage positive learning environments.

Think About . . .

What policies does your institution have in place that governs student conduct? How would you respond to a student who challenges you in a classroom setting?

Academic dishonesty can take many forms—plagiarism on written assignments, cheating on tests, buying term papers from other students, falsifying patient information and documentation, to name just a few. Many faculty are dismayed to find out that nursing students, who are studying to be professionals who are legally and ethically responsible for the lives of others, will engage in academic dishonesty while in nursing school. Some faculty consider academic dishonesty to be a personal affront to their authority as faculty. However, the stressors associated with nursing school are many, and it is indeed true that nursing students frequently engage in academic dishonesty activities for a number of reasons.

How you respond to cases of academic dishonesty will be governed by the student academic dishonesty policies in place within your institution. Student sanctions can range from receiving a "0" for the assignment to failing the course or, if serious enough such as in repeated cases of dishonest behavior, even dismissal from the institution. Review the policies so that you are familiar with the steps that need to be taken when you confront a student about suspected academic dishonesty. Seek the counsel of your immediate supervisor as well in all such incidents. Provide the student with an opportunity to address all charges before you decide upon the final sanctions.

Remaining calm, objective, and nonjudgmental is crucial in such circumstances. Students engage in such activities for a number of reasons. You have nothing to gain by taking it as a personal attack on you and becoming angry as a result. Although some students may consider academic dishonesty to be a "game" and "no big deal," for others it is an act of desperation and a significant lapse in judgment for which they are seriously repentant. It is also important that the "punishment" the student receives is befitting the "crime" that has been committed. When determining the final outcome of such a situation, rarely do you have to rush to a decision. Inform the student that you are considering all of the options available to you and that this will take some time. You can typically allow a few days to gather information from the student(s), consider the evidence, document your findings, consult authorities, and then render a decision about the sanctions that will be imposed on the student as a result. You will not regret taking the time to consider all possible outcomes before making a final decision, and as a result your decision will be more likely to be one made with thoughtfulness, clarity, and objectivity, and one that will stand up to any challenges from the student.

SETTING GOALS: THE EARLY STAGES OF YOUR TEACHING CAREER

As you begin your career as a faculty, it will be important for you to identify early stage career goals to facilitate your growth and development as a teacher. In this chapter, we have discussed what your teaching assignment may look like and how to begin to develop effective relationships with students. Chapter 2 discusses the competencies associated with facilitating learning and socialization of students, assessing and evaluating learning, and developing curricula, all of which are directly related to the teaching role. It is beyond the scope of this book, however, to provide an in-depth discussion of all of the competencies related to teaching. And it is beyond the scope of any novice faculty to focus on all of these competencies within the first year or two of teaching. Acquisition and development of the full range of competencies associated with the role of teacher comes over a period of time. Setting goals for the first 5 years of your teaching career will help you acquire these competencies in a strategic manner and ensure that you continue to grow and develop in your role as a teacher.

In the first year or two of your career as a teacher, you will want to focus on developing your "teaching presence" in the classroom and clinical setting. What characteristics do you want to develop as a teacher? Exhibit 5.1 provides you with some questions to ask yourself about what it means for you to be engaged in the teaching-learning process. Your philosophical beliefs about teaching and learning will influence the teaching strategies you use and the relationships you develop with your students. Reflecting upon your answers to these questions will help you to identify meaningful goals that you can use to shape the development of your teaching career.

In addition, as a novice teacher you can expect to focus your initial teaching goals on how to most effectively: (1) prepare lesson

Exhibit 5.1

Developing Your "Teaching Presence"

■ What philosophical beliefs do you hold about the teaching-learning process?

■ How will you demonstrate your philosophical beliefs about teaching and learning to others?

■ How will you define your role as faculty in the teaching-learning process?

■ How will you actively engage students in learning?

■ What strategies will you use to foster positive student–faculty relationships?

■ What reflective practices and evaluation strategies will you use to help you grow in the role of teacher?

plans for class or clinical learning experiences; (2) implement teaching strategies that foster active learning; (3) interact with students; (4) evaluate student learning; (5) integrate technology into your teaching; and (6) organize and manage your time to address your teaching responsibilities. Your early career plan as a teacher will benefit from setting goals in each of these areas. Having an identified teaching mentor who can assist you in setting realistic goals and identifying strategies to help you meet your goals can be very helpful.

Think About . . .

Consider each of the goal areas identified in the preceding paragraph. What are your immediate goals for developing your competence as a teacher in each of these areas? Write them down and share them with your teaching mentor.

As you become more comfortable in performing the basic competencies associated with teaching, you may wish to shift your attention to identifying areas of teaching expertise that you want to develop further as a form of scholarship. For example, have you developed a passion for identifying the most effective ways to integrate the use of technology into your teaching? Or, are you interested in seeking methods by which the integration of classroom and clinical learning experiences can be more holistically addressed for undergraduate students throughout their educational experiences? Or, are you interested in determining what models of academic–practice partnerships are most effective in aiding the transition of students from the educational environment to the practice setting? These are just a few ideas—the possibilities of where you choose to focus your scholarly interests are endless and should be driven by your own individual passions about the teaching-learning process.

If you find yourself drawn to engaging in scholarship that is related to your teaching role, then you will want to identify goals that will help you fulfill those interests. Consider what role you see the scholarship of teaching having in your academic career. Depending upon your interests and the fit for your institution, the scholarship of teaching may play a significant role in shaping your academic career. Be sure to read Chapter 6, which discusses developing as a scholar and includes a discussion on the scholarship of teaching to see if this area of scholarship is of interest to you. If this is the case, your career goals should also include goals that will lead you to eventually becoming recognized as a scholar of teaching and nursing education.

As you set your initial goals for developing your teaching, keep in mind the advice Boice (2000) provided in his book for new faculty. He stated that those faculty who are most likely to succeed in the academic environment, and indeed thrive in it, are those who practice "constancy and moderation" (p. 5) in their approach to teaching. In other words, you do not have to tackle and accomplish everything at once as you learn to become a teacher. Instead you will experience greater success and satisfaction by developing approaches to your work of teaching that allow you to pace yourself and reflect upon your teaching preparations instead of "rushing" to prepare (Boice, 2000). Teaching is indeed hard work, and the amount of effort that it takes to be successful in the classroom or clinical setting can be a surprise to new teachers. In addition, at times it may seem to you that your students are not suitably appreciative of the amount of effort that you are devoting to your teaching. To avoid frustration, burnout, and maybe even disillusionment with teaching, take the time to set your goals, and commit yourself to meeting those goals in a balanced and evenly paced approach that includes regularly scheduled time in your work schedule to prepare for teaching your courses and adequate time for reflection upon your progress as a teacher.

SEEKING RESOURCES TO DEVELOP IN THE ROLE OF TEACHER

Once you have set your teaching goals you will need to seek the resources necessary to help you meet your goals. There are a myriad number of resources in many different formats available to you to assist you in your development as a teacher. The appendix to this book contains a listing of a number of those resources. You should have no difficulty locating resources that you will find to be helpful for your particular teaching needs. These resources may take the form of institutional resources, workshops, conferences, books and journals, professional organizations, or electronic resources such as listservs and Web sites.

Institutional Resources

You should begin your search for teaching resources within your own institution. Most academic institutions offer centralized resources that are devoted to the scholarship of teaching and learning and to helping faculty develop their teaching expertise. Some schools of nursing are large enough to offer some of these same services to faculty within their school. Almost always available to faculty free of charge, these centers offer economical, individualized and easily accessible consultations with teaching and instructional design experts who will help you design your courses. There are often offices that are devoted to helping faculty integrate technology into their courses as well; for example, online learning and other forms of distance learning, the use of electronic portfolios or personal response devices ("clickers"), and computer assisted instruction, are some of the forms of technology that faculty can get assistance with adopting for use within their classrooms.

In addition to individualized assistance, these centers for teaching and learning may also offer workshops that are open only to institutional faculty and staff on a variety of teaching topics, including managing the classroom environment and dealing with academic dishonesty. Some institutions will provide internal funding in the form of grants or scholarships to assist faculty in the redesign of their courses or to support attendance at intensive weeklong teaching workshops. Be sure to inquire about the services that are provided at your particular institution and become familiar with the offerings available to you. Another benefit to using these resources is the inter-disciplinary networking that occurs when you attend workshops that are open to faculty from all disciplines. You can learn much from the experiences of other faculty who are usually very willing to share the knowledge they have gained through years of teaching.

Workshops and Conferences

In addition to the resources that are available to you within your own school and institution, be alert to conference and workshop offerings that can help you develop as a teacher.

These offerings may be local, state, regional, national, or inter-national in scope. They may be focused solely on nursing educa-tion or they may be multidisciplinary in their targeted audience. In many states, the schools of nursing will pool resources and bring the nursing faculty together for daylong workshops that are focused on a topic of general interest. You will want to investigate if such an event is offered in your state as these are typically a cost-effective means by which to engage in continuing education. Local chapters of the Sigma Theta Tau International Honor Society of Nursing and National League for Nursing's affiliated constituent leagues also may offer workshops on teaching topics of interest to you.

Other, larger venues for conferences that address issues related to nursing education include the annual National League for Nursing Education Summit, the American Association of Colleges of Nursing conferences devoted to baccalaureate, master's and doctoral educa-tion, and the biennial Sigma Theta Tau International Honor Society of Nursing Conference. Each of these conferences provides you not only with an opportunity to network with other nursing educators, but also with opportunities to publicly present your own scholarly work in nursing education. Many professional organizations also offer free or low-cost Webinars on topics that are of interest to nurse educators.

Journals and Books

In your role as a faculty, reading the current literature to stay abreast of topics and issues affecting higher education, the health professions, and nursing education is a must. You will want to set aside time in your schedule to routinely review the most recent publications. Such an investment of your time will be well worth it as you will gain access to a large body of literature that can provide you with ideas for new teaching strategies to try in your own teaching practice. There are a number of highly respected, peer-reviewed journals that are primarily dedicated to education issues. In addition, there are a significant number of education texts that are devoted to the teaching of nursing and can serve as useful reference guides for you. The appendix at the end of this book provides a listing of journals and books that you may find most helpful.

Many journals are now available online. If you do not have the resources to afford your own subscription to these journals, check out your institutional library. It is quite likely that you will have easy access to the journals through the library. Consider developing your own library of reference books that are dedicated to nursing education and other educational literature. The *American Journal of Nursing* annually publishes a list of "Books of the Year" that will contain the names of newly published books in the category of nursing education. Make it a habit to peruse this list each year to identify books that you wish to add to your personal library. The American Association of Colleges of Nursing (AACN), the National League for Nursing (NLN), and Sigma Theta Tau International (STTI) also offer publications that may be of interest to you.

Professional Organizations

Membership in professional nursing organizations is something that you will want to consider as a means of fostering your development as a teacher. Such membership can bring with it opportunities to network with other educators as well as venues through which you can disseminate your own scholarship. In addition to the organizations that have already been mentioned (the AACN, NLN, and STTI) there may be special interest groups that you will want to consider joining. For example, there are regional research groups located across the United States that provide an opportunity to come together annually within a region (e.g., Midwest Nursing Research Society, Southern Nursing Research Society, etc.) and discuss research topics of mutual interest with other nursing researchers. Most of these research societies will have a research interest group that you can join that is focused on topics of interest to nurse educators.

Electronic Resources

There are a significant number of electronic resources available that are of interest to nurse educators, and you will want to take the time to investigate this rich source of information and bookmark your favorite sites. Some of these resources are the Web sites of the prominent nursing organizations, including the American Nurses Association and the American Organization of Nurse Executives as well as AACN, NLN, and STTI. Other Web sites are devoted to higher education and focus on educational issues from a general perspective, thus being of interest to educators from all disciplines. The Carnegie Institute of the Scholarship of Teaching and Learning is an example of one such Web site. Some Web sites provide educators with teaching tools such as the Multimedia Educational Resource for Learning and Online Teaching (MERLOT) Web site, which contains free access to multidisciplinary learning objects for use in online learning. In addition, there are nurse educator listservs that can provide you with an electronic means of networking with large numbers of nurse educators who have similar questions and concerns. The appendix at the back of this book contains the Web site addresses for a number of such resources.

As you can see from this brief discussion of resources, there are many avenues by which you can seek the resources needed to assist you in developing your teaching competencies. If you are willing to invest just a little time in seeking out the resources, the benefits that you will reap will be tremendous.

Opportunities for Further Reflection

1. Think ahead 5 years—what type of teaching career do you envision for yourself? What do you need to accomplish to achieve that vision? Develop a 5-year plan that will help you meet your goals.

REFERENCES

Boice, R. (2000). *Advice for new faculty members—Nihil Nimus.* Boston: Allyn and Bacon.

Boyer, E. (1991). The scholarship of teaching from scholarship reconsidered: Priorities of the professoriate. *College Teaching, 39*(1), 11.

Clark, C. M., & Springer, P. (2010). Academic nurse leaders' role in fostering a culture of civility in nursing education. *Journal of Nursing Education, 49*(6), 319–325.

Kolanko, K., Clark, C., Heinrich, K., Serembus, J., & Sifford, K. (2006). Academic dishonesty, bullying, incivility, and violence: Difficult challenges facing nurse educators. *Nursing Education Perspectives, 27*(1), 34–43.

Luparell, S. (2007). The effects of student incivility on nursing faculty. *Journal of Nursing Education, 46*(1), 15–19.

Developing Your Identity as a Scholar

As a new faculty, one aspect of your career that you will be expected to give some consideration to is the development of your identity as a scholar. How you approach this will depend on what the scholarship expectations are within your academic institution. These expectations can vary significantly, and you will definitely want to develop an understanding of these expectations as you contemplate accepting your new position. It is essential that your own career goals for scholarship are in alignment with your institution's expectations for scholarship, or you will certainly experience frustration if you cannot comfortably align the two.

Of course, some of you might be thinking, "But I only want to teach, I don't intend to be a scholar—I can skip reading this chapter!" or "I need to focus all of my energy on teaching my students and maintaining my clinical skills—I don't have time for scholarship." Still others might be thinking, "I know that having a program of research will be necessary for me to be successful in achieving tenure, but I feel overwhelmed; how do I get my program of research started while balancing the other expectations of my role?" As you consider the extent to which being a scholar will influence your career development, one of the most important considerations for you to take away from this discussion is that all faculty, regardless of their institutional affiliation, are expected to embrace being a scholar in some form. You cannot achieve excellence in teaching or practice or both without immersing yourself in scholarly evidence and using the evidence to inform the actions you take as a teacher or a practitioner. Understanding how to develop your identity as a scholar is a crucial component of any academic career. The purposes of this chapter are to define "being a scholar," describe Boyer's model of scholarship, explore how institutional settings affect the role scholarship will play in your faculty career, identify strategies for developing as a scholar, and discuss how to seek resources to develop one's scholarship. On completion of this chapter, you should have a beginning action plan for how you will personally develop as a scholar in your faculty role.

DEVELOPING AS A SCHOLAR IN YOUR FACULTY ROLE

First, let's define what it means to be a scholar and engage in scholarship as a nurse educator. The National League for Nursing (NLN) has developed competencies for nurse educators, one of which is focused on engaging in scholarship as a nurse educator. The task statements related to the competency *Engage in Scholarship* (NLN, 2005) are listed in Chapter 2 in Exhibit 2.1. Familiarizing yourself with these task statements and reflecting on what they mean to your own educator practice is a foundational step to designing a plan that will help you develop as a scholar.

> **Think About . . .**
>
> *What does being a scholar in your faculty role mean to you? How do you think the NLN competency* Engage in Scholarship *(NLN, 2005) relates to you in your role as a nursing faculty?*

Bringing a "spirit of inquiry" to your role as an educator is the mark of a scholar. Every component of the role represents an opportunity to explore the literature and draw from previously published scholarly work to develop educational practices that are evidence-based for your own use. As the NLN (2005) competency on scholarship implies, you may have questions about active teaching strategies, student assessment or evaluation in clinical settings, "best practices" in program evaluation, teaching with technology, or the use of simulations to foster clinical decision making, to name just a few contemporary issues in nursing education. Bringing a spirit of inquiry to your practice is a wonderful habit to cultivate early in your teaching career and one that will help you stay creative, refreshed, and engaged in the role even as you become a more experienced faculty. Look around at your faculty role models—undoubtedly, you will notice that the most successful and happy in the role are those who continually ask questions of their peers and students such as, "I wonder what would happen if we tried this new approach in the classroom? Why don't we try it out and evaluate the outcomes?" Demonstrating a spirit of inquiry also means acknowledging that evaluation is a

Exhibit 6.1

How Do I Develop a "Spirit of Inquiry?"

- Keep abreast of current professional publications, within and outside the profession of nursing.
- When immersed in a new experience, identify at least one question that you want to explore more in depth to increase your understanding of the phenomena of concern.
- Network with professional colleagues, deliberately seeking out their thoughts on topics.
- Seek out individuals who hold opinions that differ from yours and genuinely consider the points of their position.
- Foster the spirit of inquiry in your students—and actively join them in searching for answers to questions to which you do not have answers.
- Commit to evaluating new teaching strategies you try so that you can learn from each experience.

key component of any teaching activity that you undertake so that you can begin to gather and analyze evaluation data that will help you determine what works and in what context, what didn't work and possible reasons as to why it didn't work, and what should any future avenues of scholarly inquiry look like? Exhibit 6.1 provides some examples of how you can develop and bring a spirit of inquiry to your role as faculty.

Growing as a scholar also means establishing an area of expertise in which you focus your scholarly efforts. How formalized you need to be in establishing your area of expertise and in what area you choose to establish yourself depend on the institutional environment in which you are working as a faculty. In institutions that have an intensive or extensive research mission, it will be very important for you to develop a specific area of expertise toward which you focus all your research, grant writing, presentations, and publications, and for you to declare that area within the first 1–2 years of your faculty appointment. Even the focus area that you choose for your research and scholarship may be directed to some extent by the research areas that the institution has decided to support with resources. In some institutions, only clinically focused research will be supported and rewarded. Other institutions may offer a broader view of scholarship and support the scholarship of teaching as well.

Four-year institutions that hold teaching to be their primary mission typically do not put as much emphasis on research productivity, but they will still expect faculty to have an area of scholarship in which they develop a reputation for expertise. These institutions are more inclined to view the scholarship of teaching as an acceptable focus for scholarly activities. Community colleges may not have formal scholarship expectations of their faculty, as their mission is strongly one of teaching excellence; however, they definitely have expectations for excellence in teaching, a goal that can be better accomplished by faculty who do develop an area of teaching expertise within the context of the community college setting. Once again, finding the right "fit" for yourself and your preferred area of scholarship is an important component of a successful academic career.

Publicly disseminating the knowledge related to the nursing discipline and the teaching of nursing, and making visible to others the outcomes of your scholarship, is another essential mark of a scholar. As a new faculty, you will want to seek out opportunities by which you can develop your presenting and writing skills. There are many ways by which you can do this, and strategies that will assist you in developing your presentation and writing skills are addressed later in this chapter. For many faculty, writing is a laborious task, one that demands discipline and concentrated time. To develop your writing skills, make a commitment to writing regularly, and find a mentor who will review your work and provide you with constructive feedback. Disseminating your scholarly work is one reason to develop your writing skills, but there are other equally important reasons for doing so. It has become increasingly important for faculty to be able to write proposals that will enable the school to develop programming or acquire resources to support teaching innovations; such writing is considered to be a form of scholarship and is an important competency to acquire.

Engaging in scholarship and developing as a scholar also require you to demonstrate the qualities of a scholar. The NLN (2005) has defined these qualities to include creativity, a sense of vitality, perseverance, courage, and of course having integrity as you go about your work as a scholar. In the next section, we explore the different types of scholarship that are typically recognized within academia so that you can gain some perspective on the wide range of scholarship conducted in academia.

DEFINING SCHOLARSHIP IN ACADEMIA

From an historical perspective, dating from the mid-19th century, scholarship within academia was originally defined as research in the traditional sense, with an emphasis on the generation and dissemination of new knowledge (Finke, 2009). Throughout the years, as research has taken on an increasingly prominent role in academia and federal funding was provided to support and encourage faculty research, the reputations of institutions of higher education became more and more tied to the research productivity of the faculty. Eventually, in many institutions, the importance of research as a gauge of the quality associated with the institution began to overshadow the importance of the teaching mission.

When nursing education transitioned from the hospital settings of diploma programs into the university settings of higher education, nursing faculty were originally at a distinct disadvantage to their faculty colleagues, from other disciplines, as coming from a practice background they did not have the same research credentials (Finke, 2009). The nursing profession struggled for many years to develop a niche in clinical research alongside other disciplines and has now reached the stage of development where prominent nurse researchers, the majority of whom are employed in academic settings, are significant contributors to research in nursing and the health professions, including medicine. In many university settings, especially academic health center institutions, it has become an expectation that nursing faculty who are seeking tenure will have a research career that includes federally funded programs of research related to clinical nursing practice.

In recent times, this traditional view of research has been broadened to include other aspects of scholarship as well, with scholarship related to teaching assuming a more prominent role within the academy. This broadening of the definition of scholarship can be traced to Boyer's (1990) work *Scholarship Reconsidered: Priorities of the Professoriate,* in which he put forth a new vision for scholarship, one that included the scholarship of teaching as well as scholarship related to other aspects of the faculty role, such as service and interdisciplinary collaboration. Boyer envisioned four forms of scholarship: the scholarship of discovery, integration, application, and teaching. Since its initial publication, this scholarship model has been used extensively in many different institutions to define and guide the development of criteria for measuring faculty scholarly productivity.

Boyer's scholarship of *discovery* is synonymous with the definition of traditional research as previously discussed in this chapter—this is scholarship that focuses on knowledge generation and dissemination. If you are interested in generating new knowledge and adding to the existing foundation of evidence-based knowledge related to any phenomena of interest, then you are engaging in the scholarship of discovery. Most of the federal funding that supports nursing research is directed toward generating new knowledge. Federal funding agencies that support the scholarship of discovery include the National Institutes of Health and the National Institutes for Nursing Research as examples. Depending on your academic institution's tenure requirements, this is the type of scholarship that you may be required to engage in to achieve promotion and tenure.

Boyer (1990) defined the scholarship of *integration* as knowledge synthesis across disciplines to address phenomena of concern, which involves bringing together discrete forms of knowledge from different contexts to create a larger, more comprehensive or holistic representation of the issue being studied. This form of scholarship is particularly meaningful in today's health care environment as we seek interdisciplinary system approaches to many of the problems that health care practitioners face in the delivery of care (Finke, 2009). Being able to work collaboratively in interdisciplinary teams to address health care concerns in complex environments will be a necessary competency for all health care providers of the future, so it is likely that we will see the scholarship of integration beginning to assume a more prominent role in the academy as well. The scholarship of integration does not replace the scholarship of discovery; rather, it is a means of integrating knowledge from different sources that has been generated through discovery.

The scholarship of *application* is related to applying what we know theoretically to address issues in practice. It is the connection of theory and practice (Finke, 2009). Nursing faculty are particularly adept at the scholarship of application, especially in the area of service learning. On many campuses, it is the nursing faculty who are leaders in developing service learning opportunities for students, in which students are immersed into a clinical setting to collaboratively provide services that the setting has identified as a priority need. To reflect the scholarship related to the application of theory to practice, it is important for faculty to identify outcomes that have been achieved as a result of student and faculty involvement in the learning activity and to disseminate those outcomes publicly through presentations and publications. Therefore, it is important for you to not be misled into thinking that this is an "easier" form of scholarship to document than the others, as it is not. It requires rigor to design, implement, and evaluate experiences that focus on application scholarship. It is most important to be able to document the process used and the theoretical foundations that guided the design and implementation of the process and report achieved outcomes related to the experiences.

Boyer's scholarship of *teaching* provides a framework by which the art and science of teaching, when built on evidence and evaluated for outcomes, is acknowledged to be a legitimate form of scholarly activity. For many nursing faculty, the scholarship of teaching is the type of scholarship that is most meaningful to their career as educators. Just being a "good" or "excellent" teacher, though, is not sufficient for the teacher to say that he or she is engaging in the scholarship of teaching. Several qualities must exist for the faculty to assert that they are engaged in the scholarship of teaching. First of all, a "spirit of inquiry" and creativity must be brought to the teaching role, whereby the teacher is constantly asking questions related to best pedagogical practices and is willing to take a risk to try new approaches in teaching and evaluate the outcomes. To engage in the scholarship of teaching, the faculty must also be willing to share the outcomes of teaching experiences with others, thus opening their teaching to peer review and critique. Sharing the outcomes of your teaching experiences with other educators also makes it possible for others to replicate what you have done in your classroom and clinical learning environments, allowing other educators to build on your work. And finally, engaging in the scholarship of teaching also means allowing for time to reflect on your teaching experiences, your successes, and your "failures," so that you can learn from each experience and apply that new knowledge to future teaching endeavors. Shulman (1998) defined the scholarship of teaching in a manner that encompasses all of these qualities when he said that the scholarship of teaching "entails a public account of some or all of the full act of teaching—vision, design, enactment, outcomes, and analysis—in a manner susceptible to critical review by the teacher's professional peers and amenable to productive employment in future work by members of that same community" (p. 6).

Think About . . .

Which forms of Boyer's (1990) scholarship are most applicable to your institutional setting? Does your institution embrace any specific scholarship model as a framework for guiding faculty scholarly activities?

DETERMINING YOUR SCHOLARSHIP "FIT"

Now that we have discussed the various forms of scholarship, as defined by Boyer, you are probably wondering "How do I know which type of scholarship is the best fit for me?" This is an important question as the answer will in large part define the type of academic career you will want to pursue. A number of factors will influence your answer to this question. These factors include your educational preparation, the type of institution within which you are employed as a faculty, the type of faculty appointment you have, and last, but *certainly not least*, your own interests and career aspirations. Because of the many factors to consider, it is important to remember that not all faculty will answer these questions in the same way, successful academic careers can take many different forms, and educational institutions typically need a diverse faculty "mix" to meet their mission. The crucial piece for you as an individual faculty is to find the "fit" that is best for you and your career aspirations. Let's look more closely at each of these factors.

Educational Preparation

Depending on the program, educational preparations can vary significantly among nursing faculty, with some faculty holding a master's degree in nursing and others holding doctoral preparation with either a research or practice degree. Your educational preparation will influence the type of scholarship that you are prepared to conduct and will also influence what your institution will expect from you. For example, for faculty holding a master's degree in nursing the institutional expectations may consist of research utilization and participation as a productive contributing member on a research team but will likely not include expectations for conducting original research (scholarship of discovery), as these are expectations of doctorally prepared faculty who hold research doctorates.

A faculty who has completed a master's degree in nursing has been prepared to draw on extant literature to review and critically appraise research, apply research findings in his or her practice, and evaluate outcomes. It is anticipated that these skills can be applied to teaching in the classroom and clinical settings, especially in the form of the scholarship of teaching. In addition, master-level graduate education also provides individuals with experiences in developing oral and written skills, so scholarship expectations may also include program development activities, proposal writing, and public dissemination of innovations related to teaching and practice activities. The scholarship of integration and application may also be applicable for faculty with master's-level preparation, especially in collaboration with others. The majority of faculty who hold the master's level of educational preparation will set personal scholarship goals that are aligned with their teaching responsibilities and their own area of clinical practice. It is not typically an expectation that you would develop a reputation for your scholarship beyond regional recognition, although this can vary from institution to institution. See Case Study 6.1 for an exemplar of how one faculty was successful in implementing personal scholarship goals in a community college setting that focus on the scholarship of teaching and are in alignment with the institution's mission of teaching excellence.

For faculty who are doctorally prepared with a research doctorate, there usually will be expectations of knowledge generation or the scholarship of discovery. Such expectations will include requirements to focus research activities in an area of expertise and to build a body of work that leads to progressively more funding, especially from external sources, to support the research activities. Usually, the research focus is a continuation of one that was previously established during your doctoral studies. Successful scholarship will be measured by your ability to establish a program of research, obtain funding to support the research, publish your work in reputable, refereed journals, and be competitively selected to present to national and international

Amy: Developing as a Scholar
in a Community College Setting

Having just graduated with her master's degree in nursing with a specialty focus in nursing education, Amy has accepted a faculty position in a statewide community college institution. Although Amy has experience as a part-time clinical instructor, this is her first full-time faculty appointment. She is eager to apply what she has learned in her graduate program to her new role as a faculty. The mission of the community college is to promote teaching excellence. As Amy begins to teach her assigned courses, she notices that her students are passive and reliant on the faculty to deliver course content. Amy begins to wonder what she might do to more fully engage her students in the classroom. She has read about using case studies and thinks this might be a teaching strategy that would be appropriate for her to try with her students. Amy discusses her ideas with the other faculty with whom she teaches. Having read about evidence-based teaching, they decide to work together to review the literature about case studies, identify evidence-based "best practices," and then design a case study scenario to implement with the students. Amy implements the scenario and evaluates the students' reaction to the strategy and their learning outcomes. At the next faculty meeting, she shares her experiences with her colleagues. Although she found some aspects of teaching with the case study to be challenging, she received feedback from her faculty colleagues and her students that she thinks will improve implementation the next time she teaches with the scenario. As she reflects on the experience, she realizes that she has initiated behaviors in her new faculty role that will help her develop as a scholar who is engaged in the scholarship of teaching.

audiences. You can see from this description that these scholarship expectations are markedly different from those previously described for those who hold a master's degree and will place different demands on your time and the scholarship goals that you set for your academic career. Case Study 6.2 illustrates how a new faculty, who is doctorally prepared and interviewing for his first academic position, selects an institution that will enable him to pursue his career goal of developing a program of research.

If you hold a practice doctorate, scholarship expectations will likely look somewhat different from the expectations described here for those who hold a research doctorate. Knowledge generation will not be an expectation, but translation of research and application to clinical or health systems issues would be an expectation consistent with the degree preparation. The scholarship of integration and scholarship of application could be particularly suited to your area of clinical expertise. In many institutions, successful scholarship will be measured by your ability to develop an identified area of clinical expertise, collaborate in interdisciplinary teams, generate proposals and support implementation of clinical care or health systems quality improvement programs, demonstrate the ability to measure and evaluate outcomes related to such programs, and disseminate the outcomes to audiences outside your institution. These expectations will lead you to develop an academic career that is different from the type of career that those with a research doctorate may have.

As you can see, your type of educational preparation does prepare you in different ways for an academic career, and developing your identity as a scholar will be shaped in part by your educational background. However, your educational preparation is just one formative piece of your scholarly identity. Your type of educational preparation may also lead you to seek employment in specific types of academic institutions, which can greatly influence the type of scholarship you will be expected to produce in your academic career. We will next discuss the influence of the academic institution on your development as a scholar.

Type of Academic Institution

Academic institutions have different expectations of faculty scholarship, and these expectations are driven by the primary mission of the institution. For example, an institution such as an academic health center that emphasizes high levels of research as a primary part of

Case Study 6.2

Paul: Developing as a Scholar in a Research Intensive University

Paul has recently completed his PhD in nursing science. His dissertation was focused on the quality of life of oncology patients. He wants to pursue an academic career that will allow him to continue to develop his program of research. As he begins his search for a faculty position, he considers what his goals are for his academic career. He knows he wants to have a position in a school that will provide him with an opportunity to teach research to undergraduate and graduate nursing students, have the infrastructure to support his development as a researcher, and provide colleagues who could mentor him in his development as a teacher and a researcher. He discusses his career goals with his faculty mentor and together they identify three schools of nursing in research universities that have programs of nursing research that closely align with his interests in quality of life in oncology patients. Next, Paul identifies some questions that he will ask during the interview process to help him determine which of these schools would be a good "fit" for the teaching and research goals he has identified. These questions include the following: How do you see my program of research fitting with the research mission of your school of nursing? Can you tell me about the research support provided to novice researchers both within the school and the university? Do you have a research mentor program? As a new teacher, do you have a program to mentor me and support my development in my teaching role? Is it possible to teach both undergraduate and graduate students? Is research a course that I could teach at both levels? Comparing the answers he receives from his interviews at the different institutions, he believes that one school is best suited to support him in his development as a researcher and teacher, and he enthusiastically accepts its offer.

its mission will have expectations of faculty that include knowledge generation and funded programs of research. Institutions that primarily offer undergraduate education are more likely to have a mission that is focused on teaching excellence and will have expectations for faculty scholarship that reflect this emphasis on teaching. Because research and scholarship expectations can vary significantly, it is crucial that you select an institution for your academic career that is most closely aligned with your own goals for scholarship and research. A poor "fit" in this area will almost assuredly lead to frustration and potential lack of success in the chosen environment, whereas a good "fit" will allow you to grow and thrive in your academic career. Given the importance of institutional fit, we describe in more detail the types of institutions and typical scholarship expectations that exist in each environment. Keep in mind that there are always exceptions to the norms that we are describing, and so it remains important for you to specifically validate the expectations of your chosen institution during the interview process.

A large percentage of basic nursing education is provided in associate degree programs that are situated in community colleges whose primary mission is providing access to quality education for diverse populations of students. Because of this educational mission, community colleges typically expect faculty to concentrate primarily on developing teaching excellence and faculty tend to carry a heavy teaching load. Faculty performance is largely evaluated and rewarded on the basis of the faculty's demonstrated proficiency in teaching and not scholarship or research. This is not to say that if you are employed as an educator in a community college setting you cannot engage in scholarship activities, but institutional resources such as grant funding and release time may not be available to support faculty scholarship development and your colleagues may not be as involved in the pursuit of such activities either. Given the emphasis on teaching excellence and the close campus–community connection community colleges have to the region they serve, you can anticipate that the scholarship of teaching and scholarship of application are the forms of scholarship that are most likely to be in evidence in such an environment.

Institutions of higher education that provide bachelor's- and master's-level educational programs often place primary emphasis on teaching excellence in their mission statements. However, because of the more comprehensive nature of their institutions they are likely to have established expectations for faculty scholarship and research as well, especially if the institutions offer graduate degrees. These expectations can vary widely from institution to institution, so you should refrain from making generalizations or assumptions about scholarship expectations. When accepting a faculty position in an institution that focuses on undergraduate or master's-level education, you will want to enquire about the degree of emphasis placed on scholarship and what types of scholarship are most valued by the institution; what faculty development and mentoring are provided to develop your scholarship skills; and, if you are seeking a tenure track appointment, how your teaching and scholarly contributions will be reviewed and evaluated for any tenure decision that is made. In some institutions, achieving tenure will be dependent on your ability to demonstrate teaching excellence as well as a certain level of scholarly productivity—teaching excellence, while expected, in and of itself will not be sufficient to achieve tenure. Ask if the institution has criteria that outline what acceptable levels of faculty scholarship look like and examine the criteria to determine your personal and professional fit with the stated expectations. Asking questions about scholarship expectations is perfectly acceptable within the interview process, and demonstrate that you have an understanding of the multiple dimensions required of the faculty role.

Institutions of higher education that have doctoral-level education and high or very high levels of research activity in their mission will have the most stringent expectations for faculty scholarship. If you wish to pursue a research-intensive academic career, you are most likely to find the best "fit" in one of these institutions. When accepting a tenure track position in a doctoral-level institution, you can expect to be offered or negotiate for "seed" funding to help you establish your program of research, a reduced teaching load to allow you more time to pursue research activities, summer support to focus on your research, and to be assigned a research mentor. In institutions that have this level of research expectation for faculty, being able to acquire internal and external funding to support your research program is important, so developing your grant writing skills will be a necessity. If grant funding is acquired that pays for your effort on the grant, you will have a reduction in your teaching load, which will allow you to direct your time toward the funded effort on the grant.

Although not necessarily a requirement, many new faculty who assume a position in a research-intensive institution have also completed a postdoctorate experience that has allowed them to further develop their research focus and skills. All forms of scholarship, as defined by Boyer, are usually acceptable in these institutions, with the scholarship of discovery receiving the highest priority. You can be expected to be told to focus your scholarship efforts in one area and develop your reputation for expertise in that area at the national and international levels. Achieving a record of publications and presentations is an absolute requirement to be successful on the tenure track. Although there is by necessity an emphasis on research and scholarly productivity, you will also be expected to achieve satisfaction in teaching and service.

As you can see by these brief descriptions of the different types of institutions and the scholarship expectations usually associated with each type, your academic career can take very different paths depending on the institution within which you choose to teach. Each setting can provide you with opportunities for a rich and rewarding career as long as the setting is aligned with what you want from your academic career, so choose your institutional environment carefully to complement all your career goals, including your goals as a nursing scholar.

Think About . . .

Which type of institution is the best "fit" for the scholarship goals you have set for yourself in your academic career? If you are uncertain about the role that scholarship and research will play in your academic career, who can you further discuss this topic with to gain additional insight into the best institutional "fit" for yourself?

Type of Faculty Appointment

In addition to educational preparation and type of institution, the type of faculty appointment you accept will influence your development as a scholar. If you accept a faculty position within a community college setting, the primary expectations for your role are going to be focused on teaching excellence. Some community colleges will offer tenure track positions, again with an emphasis on demonstrating teaching excellence, not scholarship. In contrast, most 4-year universities and colleges have multiple academic tracks for faculty appointment, with each track having its own set of unique institutional expectations related to teaching, scholarship, and service.

Regardless of the type of institution, you will want to clearly understand the set of scholarship expectations that have been developed for the track that you are appointed to, as these expectations can take many different forms. These expectations should be available to you in the faculty academic handbook or some similar document in your institution. In 4-year institutions, the two academic faculty tracks that allow for promotion in rank and are most likely to hold expectations for some form of scholarship are the tenure track and clinical track.

Tenure Track

The tenure track allows for faculty promotion within the ranks from assistant professor to associate professor and then full professor. The ultimate goal of achieving tenure, usually after 7 years on the tenure track, provides the faculty with a commitment from the institution for a permanent faculty position. Tenure track positions usually carry with them the expectation that the faculty will exhibit the competencies required to engage in research generation and dissemination and that they will gain regional, national, and eventually even international recognition for their expertise in a given focus area and the significance of the research contributions to their discipline.

On the tenure track, engaging in scholarship will typically include writing grants to attract funding (internal and external) to support your *focused* program of research as well as publishing your findings in refereed journals and being competitively selected to present your findings at professional conferences. Being able to attract grant funding, becoming published, and being selected to present are external forms of recognition regarding the value of your work and are typically considered to be the minimal set of scholarship requirements for achieving tenure within an institution. However, the *extent* to which you would need to demonstrate these accomplishments on the tenure track will be institutionally dependent.

For example, if you are developing a program of research related to the quality of life for patients with end-stage renal failure and you hold a faculty position in a small, liberal arts college, you might be expected to write some smaller local or regional grants that will fund a pilot study of your research, present your findings at local, state, and regional conferences with some national presentations in evidence, and publish as author or coauthor refereed manuscripts that are content based, as well as some that are data based. If you are pursuing the same line of research on the tenure track in an academic health center, the research expectations will likely include that you secure a series of significant and consistent grant funding that leads to external funding from federal agencies, an emerging reputation on the national level as evidenced by a number of refereed research-based presentations at national conferences, and an average of two published manuscripts a year with you as primary author with an emphasis on publishing data-based (research) articles. These two broad examples demonstrate how very different institutional expectations can be for the same track—the tenure track—across the different types of academic institutions. Having an understanding for yourself about how much emphasis you will want to place on the research component of your academic career is crucial so that you can seek out a faculty position in an institution that is in alignment with your goals.

Clinical Track

In addition to a tenure track, some institutions have a clinical track for faculty who have specific areas of clinical expertise with the primary expectation that faculty on the clinical track will share their clinical expertise with students through instruction in the practice setting. The clinical track may or may not be tenure eligible. The research or scholarship expectations for clinical track faculty will again be variable across institutions, but generally speaking, the expectations will be more closely aligned to scholarship that involves the application of evidence-based practices to clinical care or the scholarship of teaching in the practice setting.

If you accept a clinical track appointment, you can anticipate your primary workload to be related to teaching. Scholarship expectations may consist of, as examples, such activities as participating in clinical research teams to apply research findings to specific patient populations, developing quality improvement processes to improve patient care, working in interdisciplinary, collaborative teams to develop a patient safety curriculum and publishing the outcomes of the project, or developing innovative ways to instruct nursing and health professions students in the practice setting. Although these are just a few examples of scholarship activities meant to illustrate how scholarship can be related to the clinical practice role, you can see that such scholarship takes a very different form from the more traditional research expectations that were described for faculty on the tenure track. The clinical track allows you to blend your clinical expertise with your teaching expertise, and to engage in scholarship that helps to bridge the gap between education and practice with the ultimate goal of improving patient care.

Think About . . .

What type of faculty appointment do you have or are you seeking? Have you familiarized yourself with the research and scholarship expectations related to your faculty appointment? Does your institution and/or school have written expectations about research and scholarship for you to review?

In Pursuit of Your Own Scholarship Interests

We have discussed how your educational preparation, type of institution, and type of faculty appointment will influence your development as a nursing scholar. What we have not discussed is the importance of defining your own scholarship interests and developing a plan to pursue these interests. First and foremost, you must understand where your passion for research and scholarship lies. Is it in the generation of new knowledge or finding innovative ways to translate research knowledge into practice? Is it in the investigation of clinical issues or educational issues?

Do you see research playing a primary and dominant role in your academic career or a more secondary role to the pursuit of teaching excellence? If you envision an academic career that is built on a research emphasis, have you given some thought to the area in which you will focus your research? If you already hold a doctoral degree, you have already made some preliminary decisions about this when you conducted your dissertation research, as the dissertation is often used to lay the initial foundation for future research. Is this an area that will yield potential funding opportunities? Is there a school of nursing that has already developed a cadre of researchers with expertise in your chosen area, where you can seek mentorship and further development in the researcher role? These last two questions are very important as schools must consolidate their resources around areas of focused research strength that are fundable so that they can provide adequate support for faculty researchers and develop quality graduate education programs designed to produce future researchers. If your program of research is not viewed as a "fit" for the institution, you will not be likely to have a satisfying academic career within the school.

If you do not envision research as having a dominant role in your career, you will still want to consider how you will contribute to the scholarship of teaching in the classroom and clinical settings. As stated at the beginning of this chapter, all educators have the responsibility to embrace scholarship to some extent to remain current and relevant in their teaching role. So give some thought about where *your* particular scholarly interests lie and the type of institutional environment that will most likely foster the further development of these interests.

What should you do if you are saying to yourself, "I am really unsure about how best to focus my research and scholarly interests?" A first step is to schedule time to have a conversation with your chairperson or mentor about this topic. Discussing your scholarly interests with an experienced faculty member who has been successful in establishing a record of research or scholarship, especially in your institution, can be very helpful. Following such a discussion, sitting down and creating an action plan for developing your program of research and scholarship that you review annually will help you stay focused and on track.

EARLY CAREER STRATEGIES FOR DEVELOPING AS A SCHOLAR

Let's discuss how you can create an action plan for your development as a scholar and the types of experiences you will want to include in your plan. Scholarship development will usually include the following: developing an area of focus for your scholarship; developing your skills as a presenter and as a writer so that you can further develop and disseminate your ideas; and furthering your expertise in your area of scholarship. Any plan that you develop should address each of these areas.

We have already discussed the importance of having a focused area of research or scholarship and that this area may be a clinical area of interest or a teaching area of interest. Immerse yourself in the literature and become familiar with the state of the science related to your chosen focus area. Connect with leading researchers who have focused on your area of interest and become familiar with their work. You can do this at your own school or university, through attendance at regional or national research conferences, or through individual contacts. Most established researchers welcome the opportunity to discuss their program of research with others who are interested in studying the same phenomena. You may also wish to ask other faculty colleagues, either at your institution or another institution, to join you and form research teams or interest groups to explore common areas of inquiry—this can be an especially productive approach in institutions that have less developed research infrastructures or in which the faculty have significant teaching loads yet must also meet expectations for scholarship.

Identify potential gaps in knowledge related to your chosen research interest, either from your own studies or others, and develop inquiry questions that will lead to the development of research studies. Set realistic goals for writing research proposals that will help you acquire funds to pursue your research. Seek consultation for your ideas and review of your grants—remember that developing your scholarship program should not be an isolated effort but one in which you draw on the experience and support of those who have the expertise to mentor you.

Another priority in your development as a scholar is to cultivate the writing skills necessary to write grant proposals to acquire funds for research and other initiatives, as well as abstracts and manuscripts that will allow you to disseminate your work to others. Writing takes time, practice, and patience and is best accomplished by scheduling regular times on your calendar in which you are able to write for uninterrupted intervals. Failure to schedule time for writing will result in failure to write. Boice (2000) provided a series of writing tips that are helpful for novice writers to incorporate into their routine, including suggestions of writing before you are ready, writing on a regular basis, and practicing moderation in your writing sessions. Work with your mentor to identify potential writing projects, learn to seek and accept constructive critique of your writing, and strive to develop writing habits that will serve you well throughout your academic career.

Honing your presentation skills is another priority for your development as a scholar. Start by presenting your work to your colleagues within your school and campus, and seeking out regional- or state-level opportunities to present. Talk to more experienced faculty and ask them for tips on how to prepare effective presentations. Many novice presenters have also found it valuable to assemble a group of colleagues to do a "mock" presentation with them first, to perfect the pace and timing of the presentation.

Continuing to develop your expertise in your area of scholarship can be accomplished in a number of ways. Attendance at workshops and conferences is one method. Volunteering to serve as a reviewer of abstracts and manuscripts in your area of expertise is another. Joining research interest groups and committees are the other ways to expose yourself to diverse ways of thinking and keeping up to date on emerging topics in your field. Seek the advice of your chair or mentor to help you decide which of these activities are most appropriate in which for you to engage.

SEEKING RESOURCES TO DEVELOP AS A SCHOLAR

As a new faculty, you will find it beneficial to access the resources made available to you by your institution to help you adjust to your new role. Most institutions provide new faculty with a series of orientation sessions designed to address the various components of your faculty role, including your development as a scholar. Grant writing workshops, conduct of research workshops offered by the institutional review board of your institution, and writing for publication workshops are just a few examples of the type of resources that are typically freely available to faculty. Attend any workshops offered by your school or institution that provides a review of tenure and promotion guidelines and be sure to familiarize yourself with the institution's scholarship expectations. Using these guidelines to develop a trajectory for your development as a scholar will help ensure your success at your institution.

Many institutions provide small internal funding opportunities to help you launch your program of research or other scholarly projects. Seek these opportunities and take advantage of them—they may be available from your school, institutional centers devoted to the scholarship of teaching, research departments, and other sources.

Professional organizations will also offer funding opportunities for new investigators. The message for you to take away from this discussion is that it pays for you to be vigilant in scanning your environment for development opportunities and to take full advantage of these resources to help you in your development.

Opportunities for Further Reflection

1. Reflect on what you have read in this chapter and how it applies to your career aspirations as a scholar. Develop a 1- to 2-year plan for your own scholarly development that is appropriate for your academic institution's environment. Share this plan with your mentor.

REFERENCES

Boice, R. (2000). *Advice for new faculty members*. Boston: Allyn & Bacon.

Boyer, E. (1990). *Scholarship reconsidered: Priorities of the professoriate*. Princeton, NJ: The Carnegie Foundation for the Advancement of Teaching.

Finke, L. (2009). Teaching in nursing: The faculty role. In D. M. Billings & J. A. Halstead (Eds.), *Teaching in nursing: A guide for faculty* (3rd ed., pp. 3–17). St. Louis, MO: Saunders Elsevier.

National League for Nursing. (2005). *Core competencies for nurse educators*. New York: Author.

Shulman, L. (1998). Course anatomy: The dissection & analysis of knowledge through teaching. In Pat Hutchings (Ed.), *The course portfolio: How faculty can improve their teaching to advance practice and improve student learning*. Washington, DC: American Association of Higher Education.

Determining Your Service Commitment

Modern nursing has a strong heritage of service. From Florence Nightingale to nurses in our own era who do disaster relief, nurses are among the first to volunteer when needed. This need to serve carries over into our academic careers. Service is one of the components of the tripartite academic mission of most higher education institutions and is expected of all faculty. In fact, one of the competencies of the National League for Nursing (NLN) Core Competencies of Nurse Educators (2005) is *Function as a Change Agent and Leader.* This competency speaks to the faculty member's service role and the importance of providing leadership and service to one's academic institution, as well as the profession (Halstead, 2007). One of the ways that you can function as a change agent and leader is through various forms of service. In addition, service opportunities may provide a way for you to integrate your role as a clinician with your teaching and scholarly roles (Nardi & Wilson, 2008).

Before becoming a faculty member, you may have served on committees in your workplace and in professional and community organizations. As a graduate student, you may have been a student representative on a faculty search committee or a student representative on one or more governance committees at your school. These experiences have helped shape your career to date and will serve you well as you progress in your career. The transition to the role of new faculty member requires you to rethink the role that your service commitments will play in your career development. You will be expected to have service accomplishments that are relevant to your institution, community, profession, and your own area of expertise.

One word of caution, however, is that it can be very easy to become overextended in your service commitments. You will need to learn how to consider carefully all the available service opportunities that are offered to you. You can say "yes" to those that are most meaningful to you and your career, and "no" to those that do not appear to have any "value-added" benefits for you professionally or personally.

Sometimes, you will need to know when it is your "turn" to provide service to your school, not because it will be particularly meaningful to you, but because it is part of being a good "citizen" of the academy. Doing your share contributes to a productive work environment.

Therefore, the purpose of this chapter is to define the various types of service commitments that you will be asked to consider and explore how these commitments fit into the totality of your academic career. Although Chapter 8 will give you an outline of the entire first years of your career and show you how to make career plans long-term, this chapter will specifically focus on choosing appropriate service commitments in the early part of your career.

WHAT IS SERVICE?

Broadly speaking, service is sharing your talents in meaningful ways with the educational institution, the profession, and the community. The first 1 or 2 years as a faculty member, your service commitments generally will be light, because you will be focusing on your teaching role and scholarship. After you have established yourself in your faculty role, service will take up about 10% to 15% of your faculty load. However, if you are certified, your service commitment may be more in the range of 20% as one of the ways you maintain your certification is through active clinical practice.

Although all institutions expect service from faculty, how they value and reward service varies significantly. When considering the types of service commitments you might want to make, you will want to make sure that you understand how your institution figures service into your total workload and also how the institution views service when considering tenure and promotion decisions, if you are on the tenure track. For example, some institutions give faculty members 1 day a week, or approximately 20% of total workload for scholarship and service combined, including clinical practice. In other institutions, clinical practice and scholarship are figured as separate entities when total workload is configured.

In major research universities, community service may be the least valued aspect of your faculty performance. However, a university that has a community engagement mission will place more value on professional and community service. Indeed, the Carnegie Classification of Institutions of Higher Education has an elective classification of Community Engagement. The Carnegie Foundation for the Advancement of Teaching (2010) states that community engagement is "the collaboration between institutions of higher education and their larger communities (local, regional/state, national, global) for the mutually beneficial exchange of knowledge and resources in a context of partnership and reciprocity" (Carnegie Foundation for the Advancement of Teaching, paragraph 3).

Through these activities, faculty participate in the scholarship of community engagement. According to Boyer (1996), the scholarship of application includes community engagement. One way faculty participate in the scholarship of community engagement is by incorporating service learning initiatives, which we will discuss later in this chapter, into their courses.

As you can see, universities define and value service in different ways. The same holds true for community colleges. Service commitments usually address the following areas: service to the institution (program and campus), service to the discipline, and service to the community through community engagement. Institutions will expect you to demonstrate service in each of these areas. In addition, as you gain experience in your faculty role and move toward achieving tenure and promotion, expectations increase. Thus, you should gradually expand your service contributions from the local venue to national and even international levels.

Another important component of your service commitments is being able to document the outcomes that have occurred as a direct result of your participation and leadership in service efforts. It is not enough to simply state that you were a member of a committee or task force, or that you chaired or led an initiative; you will need to be able to demonstrate what was achieved as a result of your contributions. We will discuss each of the different areas of service in more detail.

Academic Service

Service within the university is the most basic level that is expected and is the mark of good academic citizenship (Krothe & Warner, 2007). Academic citizenship involves not only being respectful of your colleagues by learning how to negotiate differences in views when making, for example, decisions regarding curriculum revision, but also participating in committees and other work groups. All faculty have a stake in decisions made by committees; therefore, all faculty should participate in those committees making the decisions. Of course, you must balance the level of participation you seek with the rest of your faculty workload demands.

Typically, by the second year of your faculty appointment, you should be on at least one departmental committee, and by the third year you will want to seek membership on one university committee. As mentioned previously, however, it is important to clarify the specific service expectations for your program and institution. Some departments expect that you will have taken on a leadership role on committees by your third year of appointment. Other departments may not expect you to assume a leadership role until your fourth or fifth year.

Unfortunately, in many institutions the burden of committee work and leadership often falls to the more junior faculty because they "need" to demonstrate service. Junior faculty may be afraid to say "no" to a request for service as they wish to be seen as contributing members to the team and fear retribution in some manner if they decline an opportunity to serve. For every opportunity to serve that you accept, you will want to be able to articulate not only what your participation will mean to the department or institution but also what your participation will mean to you in your own professional growth and development.

There are several things for you to consider prior to choosing your service commitments. First, you will want to understand the service opportunities that are available to you in your program and institution and the nature of these opportunities. There will usually be a number of standing committees (as determined by the bylaws of the program and institution) and there will likely to be a number of task forces as well. Serving on a standing committee usually implies a term time commitment, which may be as long as 2 to 3 years. Task forces are usually formed to address a particular issue and are time limited in nature, disbanding once the charge to it has been met. Some committees may meet regularly on a monthly basis, while others only meet one or two times a year to perform their functions. Task forces, although time limited, may need to meet frequently on an intensive schedule to complete their charge. You might also inquire if the committee members choose the meeting times. If the time is preset, your classroom and clinical teaching schedule might conflict with the set time.

Second, you will want to know how participation on committees and task forces is decided. This is usually decided in one of three ways: through appointment, by election, or by soliciting volunteers. Your department chair or dean can help provide this information to you. Some committees may also require that the faculty participants have tenured status. For example, volunteering for a curriculum committee may be sufficient to place you on the committee. However, most personnel committees, such as faculty affairs, promotion and tenure, and grievance committees, will require tenure for membership. Some college or division-wide committee memberships may be determined at the department level through an election or volunteer selection.

Third, you will need to know the functions or duties of the committees that you are considering joining. Do these duties match your interest or expertise? Alternatively, will participation in the committee work foster your professional growth and development in the faculty role by providing you with experiences that you have not yet had?

Service at the institutional level comes about in several ways. If there is a university senate or faculty council, election to the body is the norm. Various academic units on campus elect members to this body. Whether membership on a faculty senate requires tenure is variable. If tenure is not required, and your department and you value service on the senate, you might consider running for senate in your fourth or fifth year of your faculty appointment.

Oftentimes the senate or council, or a subset of this body, will make appointments to the university-wide committees from a pool of volunteers. Be alert for the calls for membership on the various committees if institution-wide service is an expectation.

While university service does take time, the benefits can outweigh the time spent. You will meet other faculty from across campus; you can give the nursing program a voice on committees; and you can get an important view of the issues from a campus-wide perspective. One word of caution, however: If you are a member of an underrepresented group, you may be asked to be on numerous committees because committees seek to have diverse memberships. Members of underrepresented groups do need to have a major voice in academic decision making. However, do not feel obligated to say yes to everything! Similar to our advice above, select your participation based on your expertise and interest. Saying yes too often will lead you to a life that leaves little time for personal ventures.

Considering the various forms of academic service to be involved in can be overwhelming. When you look at Exhibit 7.1, determine the levels of service that are available at your school. Not all the types of service are present at each educational institution. However, you can use this list to help you make sense of available academic service opportunities.

Exhibit 7.1

Examples of Academic Service Opportunities

Program-Level Service

Undergraduate Curriculum Committee
Graduate Curriculum Committee
Student Affairs Committee
Faculty Affairs Committee

Institutional-Level Service

Faculty Senate
Graduate Council
Academic Integrity Committee
Speakers Series Committee
Graduation Committee
Athletics Committee
Institutional Review Board

Never underestimate the value of good academic citizenship. Your contributions to the workings of the organization are important. Faculty participation in decision making is a hallmark of effective academic organizations.

Think About . . .

What type of academic service interests you and is a good "fit" for your expertise? What type of service expectations are required at your institution?

Professional Service

Professional service is service that uses your talents to benefit the nursing profession and health professions, in general, including the nursing and higher education communities. Professional service comes in various forms. Committee membership and leadership and serving as a reviewer of abstracts, textbooks, and manuscripts are just some of the ways you can provide professional service. We will discuss each of these in more detail.

Committee Work

Committee work as an active member or an officer in a professional organization is common. Most faculty initially become involved in local organizational work as one means by which to begin to contribute service to the profession. Some of the professional organizations that are most likely to have local chapters in your region include Sigma Theta Tau International Honor Society of Nursing, NLN constituent leagues, American Organization of Nurse Executives, state nurses associations, nursing research societies, and specialty nursing organizations, such as those dedicated to critical care nursing, oncology nursing, or advanced practice nursing, to name just a few.

For example, one way to get started in professional service is to be on a committee or run for office in your local Sigma Theta Tau chapter. Your service at the chapter level may provide you with an opportunity to attend the Biennial International convention, where you will meet others who have similar scholarly and service interests. As you use your local chapter leadership experiences to network nationally and internationally, you are developing contacts. These contacts might lead to future opportunities for service at the national or international level.

As previously mentioned, service can also involve working with local chapters of specialty nursing organizations. Providing service to a specialty organization may provide a good venue for you to combine your scholarship and service interests. One way to do this is to present some of your scholarly work during a local meeting. Combining service with scholarly activities is always a good idea! Local presentations can serve as rehearsals for presentations at national meetings.

At the state level, service through your state nurses' association or a constituent league of the NLN provides venues for professional service. Specialty organizations also have state organizations in which you can serve on committees and make presentations.

Peer Reviewer

Committee membership and leadership are not the only ways to give service to the profession. Many opportunities exist for peer review

Case Study 7.1

Linda: Second-Year Faculty Member
at a Major Research University

Linda is a faculty member at a major research university. During her first year on faculty, she made two research presentations: one at a regional research conference and another at a national meeting. In the packets of materials at both meetings were calls for peer reviewers for abstract submissions. Linda volunteered to review for the regional research organization, and at the end of her second year as a faculty member, the regional organization asked her to submit her CV as a precursor to being chosen as an abstract reviewer. She continued as an abstract reviewer for several years, then, through her contacts with the national organization where she presented her research, she became a manuscript peer reviewer for a nursing research journal. In summary, she had heeded the call of the coordinator of new faculty orientation, who stated, "Don't focus on service during your first year; wait, and start slow in your second year." Linda did that, and each year beginning in her second year as a faculty member, she gradually added more service commitments. Linda expanded her commitments beyond the regional level to include service at the national level.

---

of manuscripts submitted for publication, review of grant proposals submitted for funding, and abstracts submitted for conference presentations. One important benefit of peer reviewing is the opportunity to see what others are doing in your area of scholarly interest.

How do you get to be a peer reviewer? Linda in Case Study 7.1 is a good example of a faculty who establishes contacts that eventually lead to her becoming a reviewer.

Notice how she has capitalized on her contacts at professional meetings. How might you use your attendance at professional meetings to combine your scholarly skills with service to a professional organization?

Contacts with textbook salespersons at national and regional meetings and at the local level during sales calls can lead to opportunities to review book chapters and supporting teaching materials, such as test banks, for upcoming books. Before textbooks are published, sample chapters and other materials are sent to reviewers for critique. Moreover, even before textbooks are written, publishers will sometimes send out the prospectus, or publication proposal, to reviewers to see if a market exists for the textbook. Publishers usually pay a small honorarium for such reviews.

More experience in peer reviewing conference abstracts, grants, and articles can lead to membership on editorial boards of journals. These boards set the journal's direction with regard to the nature of the articles that the journal publishes. Editorial board members also serve as peer reviewers for the prospective articles. One thing to note about peer reviewing, however, is that you can become so involved in peer review activities that you have little time for your own scholarship.

Having the opportunity to serve at the national level takes a concerted networking effort for others to know you. Attending conferences is the best way to make national contacts. At these conferences, talk with people before and after the sessions. If you are attending a meeting with a more senior faculty member from your school, ask to be introduced to others who are attending the meeting. After attending several conferences and conventions, you will begin to see familiar faces. Your network will grow larger and you will have more opportunities to volunteer for service.

What meetings will you attend? Gordon's experiences, which are described in Case Study 7.2, show how sustained attendance at meetings can lead to service at the national level. Notice how he chose his service to match his interests.

Clinical Practice as Service

Clinical practice is another way faculty engage in professional service. Many faculty, particularly those who are advanced practice nurses, practice 1 day a week and in the summer months. If your teaching duties include clinical teaching, keeping up your clinical skills is essential. Some faculty keep up their skills through the teaching itself, but many desire to maintain an active clinical practice. Not only does practice maintain clinical skills but it also helps faculty obtain and maintain specialty certification.

One challenge, however, is to fit clinical practice into a hectic faculty schedule. During the academic year, unless practice is figured formally into your faculty load, you may find that maintaining an

---

Case Study 7.2

Gordon: A Community College Faculty Member

Gordon teaches full-time at a community college. He has attended a professional development meeting for associate degree faculty for several years. During these meetings, he has attended a number of sessions on community-based education. While at these sessions, he talked with meeting participants and subsequently communicated with them via e-mail. As a result, when a call went out for membership on a task force on community-based education, he volunteered and was chosen to serve. After several more years of active involvement on this and various other task forces, the organization nominated Gordon to run for office.

---

active practice will be difficult. Most institutions will allow faculty to practice a maximum of 1 day a week. If you wish to practice more often than that, you will need to negotiate an arrangement with your department chair or dean. Sometimes, however, you can also integrate your faculty practice with your clinical teaching. For example, if you are a nurse practitioner or clinical nurse specialist, you can precept graduate students as you see your clients.

Think About . . .

Will you maintain a clinical practice? If so, how will you integrate practice into your schedule?

Some nursing programs have faculty practice plans. These plans exist in several variations. Schools may run nurse-managed clinics where faculty and students see clients, who pay for the services offered. The school keeps any profits earned. The school may use the earned profits to support faculty development, defray part of the cost of the faculty salaries, or purchase equipment. In some faculty practice models, faculty are contracted to deliver services to outside agencies and the faculty and school may each gain a share of the salary earned. In another model, a school sets up a consulting service wherein faculty consult with organizations on a full range of direct and indirect care issues and both faculty and school reap the rewards (Miller, Bleich, Hathaway, & Warren, 2004). Faculty may also serve as independent contractors in clinical agencies. In this model, the faculty member keeps all the salary earned. In all of these models, faculty may integrate teaching with service.

Faculty practice provides an environment rich with opportunities to integrate scholarship with practice. For instance, faculty and students can develop a research project with the purpose of testing a nursing intervention on clients served. Data from the health records can be analyzed for patterns of health behaviors.

Think About . . .

What ways can you integrate teaching, scholarship, and service to maximize your energy and enrich the faculty roles in which you engage?

Faculty practice also comes in the various forms of consultation. For example, you can provide consultation for a hospital that is conducting evidence-based practice projects. Alternatively, you can provide consultation regarding various nursing administration or nursing education issues.

Another form of consultative faculty practice can be in the form of membership on committees at a health care agency. For instance, you could serve as a consultant to a quality improvement committee or an evidence-based practice committee. Your consultation focus will be based on your areas of expertise.

One thing to note is that your educational institution may have regulations that limit the time you can devote to paid consultation. Most schools allow 1 day a week for consultation during the academic year. Usually, during the summer, you are free to work for pay as much as you desire. Those on 12-month contracts are most likely bound by the 1-day-a-week rule year-round.

The reason the institution limits outside work is that your main loyalty is to your primary employer. If you are away from campus multiple days a week for personal gain, you are unavailable for students who wish to meet with you outside of scheduled class and clinical times. Furthermore, you are not available for university service, which enhances your academic citizenship.

Some faculty may also want to supplement their salary with teaching an additional course online or in person for another institution. Again, you may have to seek permission from your primary employer. Some institutions may allow this practice and others may interpret teaching for another nursing program as a conflict of interest.

Exhibit 7.2 summarizes the diverse opportunities for professional service. Consider which forms of professional service interest you and capitalize on your talents. In addition, reflect about the methods of service that allow you to integrate teaching and scholarship.

Community Service

You will also be expected to provide service to your community. The extent to which the community service will be expected and the type of community service that is acceptable will vary with the organization. Community service, generally speaking, is any community activity in which a faculty member participates. However, for community service to be considered and evaluated for promotion and tenure efforts, the community service usually has to be related in some manner to the faculty member's professional expertise. For example, providing health education at a homeless shelter capitalizes on your professional expertise. Some institutions do keep track of such things as a faculty member's participation in community theater, scouting, or religious education. These kinds of activities show how the academic organization contributes to the community at large. However, these same institutions rarely count these activities for promotion and tenure unless they are directly applied to the faculty's area of expertise.

For example, a nursing faculty's involvement in establishing a faith-based, parish nursing program at his or her church would be considered to be a form of community service as it capitalizes on the faculty's professional expertise. Alternatively, you could use your nursing background to serve on a United Way funding panel or be a member of the board for a nonprofit organization that helps women

Exhibit 7.2

Examples of Selected Professional Service Opportunities

National Nursing Organizations

American Association of Colleges of Nursing—
http://www.aacn.nche.edu
American Association of Nurse Executives—
http://www.aone.org/
American Nurses Association—http://www.nursingworld.org/
National League for Nursing—http://www.nln.org/
Sigma Theta Tau International—http://www.nursingsociety
.org/

Specialty Nursing Organizations

American Academy of Nurse Practitioners—
http://www.aanp.org/
American Association of Critical Care Nurses—
www.aacn.org
Association of Women's Health, Obstetrics, and Neonatal
Nursing—http://www.awhonn.org/
National Association of Clinical Nurse Specialists—
http://www.nacns.org/
Oncology Nursing Society—http://www.ons.org/

Examples of Other Forms of Service

Membership on clinical agency committees
Conducting workshops for clinical agencies

and children who have been victims of domestic violence. Exhibit 7.3 illustrates examples of community service in which nursing faculty often participate.

Another important type of community service is through engaging your students in service learning. Although many campuses promote service learning, universities that have a community and civic

---

Exhibit 7.3

**Examples of Community Service Opportunities
(all these provide service learning opportunities)**

Fund raising for nonprofit organizations
Providing care at homeless shelters, free clinics, and domestic
abuse shelters
Faith-based nursing
Organizing influenza immunizations for a county health
department
Planning a health fair for a senior citizens' center
Board member for a nonprofit organization

---

engagement mission often place a special emphasis on service learning throughout the various curricula on campus. Service learning is predicated on the notion that faculty facilitate opportunities that foster social responsibility and civic engagement in their students (Mueller & Billings, 2009). The goal is for students to help improve the world in which they live.

Institutions classified as community engagement institutions have curricula that promote student and faculty work with their communities. Through service learning activities, all parties to the engagement benefit. The community works with members of the academic community to plan a service, and as a result faculty and student scholarship benefit. If the institution also emphasizes outreach to the community, the campus uses its resources to collaborate with the community on such things as economic development. Again, both parties to the partnership benefit (Carnegie Foundation for the Advancement of Teaching, 2010).

You might think service learning is just another name for clinical experiences or volunteering. However, service learning is much more than that. In fact, clinical experiences are not necessarily considered a form of service learning, unless key features are evident in the learning experience. One such key feature of service learning is working in a community to solve a *community-identified* problem. One outcome of service learning is to promote citizenship responsibilities

Case Study 7.3

Fund Raising for the March of Dimes

As part of a freshman introduction to health professions course, students had an academic requirement to learn about a health issue in the community. A group of students, under the direction of the instructor, worked with the March of Dimes to plan a fund-raising walk. These students were to hand out pamphlets at the walk and answer questions about how to decrease the rate of premature births. Students researched the causes of prematurity and learned about ways to decrease the rate of premature births. On the day of the walk, the students staffed the education booth along with their instructor. They provided education to a number of walkers. During the debriefing following the day of the walk, many students commented that they had known little about prematurity until their participation in this activity.

(Mueller & Billings, 2009). One example of a service learning project would be students working with a nonprofit organization to plan a fundraiser for that organization. Case Study 7.3 illustrates the benefits of service learning. When looking at this case, you will see that students learned about the scope of the health problem involved and the agency benefited from the funds raised.

WHAT TO DO?

As stated at the outset of this chapter, the service component of your faculty role is important, but it does not receive as much emphasis in your faculty role as do teaching and scholarship. So how do you decide how much time to devote to your service efforts? The answer to this question depends on your academic institution's expectations. However, one thing is for certain: Service is rarely a substitute for good teaching and fulfilling scholarly expectations. In fact, Kaufman (2007), reporting on the NLN/Carnegie Foundation Survey "Nurse Educators: Compensation, Workload, and Teaching Practices," showed that nursing faculty work more than 53 hours per week. According to Kaufman's summary of this study, three-fourths of faculty time is devoted to student contact. Other time is divided among clinical practice (7%), academic service (7.2%), and research (5.6%). The rest of the time is devoted to administrative duties (Kaufman, 2007, pp. 296–297). Certainly, these numbers vary with the type of institution and teaching assignment. For instance, those who teach in graduate programs spend more time on scholarship. Nevertheless, what is clear is that service commitments can prevent you from developing your scholarship.

As stated before, synergistically combining roles, whenever possible, is one of the keys to survival in the academic environment. Moreover, just as important, you must know your academic institution's expectations with regard to service. Academic institutions expect to benefit from your professional and community service. If you are elected to a national office, your name is attached to your institution and the institution garners recognition from your election. The institution might use that recognition to attract new faculty and students. Likewise, if your students engage in a service learning activity, the community will come to value your institution. As a result, stakeholders, such as legislators, might advocate for funding for the academic institution as well as the community. Community engagement and service learning are wonderful ways for academic institutions to bridge the "town–gown" gap. Doing so garners much support for the institution, and students and communities benefit in the end.

Service is an essential part of good academic, professional, and community citizenship. However, service commitments cannot over shadow your other responsibilities without prior agreement with your institution. In special cases, as you develop in your career, you may have a major service responsibility that results in a lighter teaching load or deferral of scholarly expectations. In those rare cases in which a faculty member is elected to a major office in a national organization, workload expectations may be adjusted. The same might hold true for faculty who chair the institution-wide faculty organization. Nevertheless, this kind of arrangement rarely happens early in your career.

Leadership is an essential nurse educator competency (Halstead, 2007). Service provides an opportunity to demonstrate your leadership capabilities and to promote required change in the academic organization, the profession, and the community.

Opportunities for Further Reflection

1. What talents do I have that I can use to provide service to the academic institution, the profession, and the community?
2. How will I decide where to serve?

REFERENCES

Boyer, E. L. (1996). The scholarship of engagement. *Journal of Public Service and Outreach, 1*(1), 11–20.

Carnegie Foundation for the Advancement of Teaching. (2010). *Classification description: Community engagement elective classification.* Retrieved May 24, 2010, from http://classifications.carnegiefoundation.org/descriptions/community_engagement.php

Halstead, J. A. (2007). *Nurse educator competencies: Creating an evidence-based practice for nurse educators.* New York: National League for Nursing.

Kaufman, K. (2007). More findings from the NLN/Carnegie National Survey. *Nursing Education Perspectives, 28,* 296–297.

Krothe, J. S., & Warner, J. R. (2007). Perceptions of tenured nursing faculty related to decision-making for community service. *Nursing Outlook, 55,* 202–207.

Miller, K. L., Bleich, M. R., Hathaway, D., & Warren, C. (2004). Developing the academic nursing practice in the midst of new realities in higher education. *Journal of Nursing Education, 43,* 55–59.

Mueller, C., & Billings, D. M. (2009). Service learning: Developing values and social responsibilities. In D. M. Billings & J. A. Halstead (Eds.), *Teaching in nursing: A guide for faculty* (3rd ed.). St. Louis, MO: Saunders/Elsevier.

Nardi, D., & Wilson, C. (2008). A faculty practice plan for the acute and critical care nurse. *AACN Advanced Critical Care, 19*(1), 78–84.

National League for Nursing. (2005). *Core competencies of nurse educators.* Retrieved May 29, 2010, from http://www.nln.org/facultydevelopment/pdf/corecompetencies.pdf

Planning Your Career Trajectory

Obtaining an academic position is, of course, just the first step in your successful career. You must make a conscious effort to plan your career pathway. Mary McKinney (2010), an academic coach, advocated making a 6-year plan. Why is a 6-year plan a first step in career planning? Six-year plans get you ready for that first benchmark: tenure. New faculty members are usually appointed at the assistant professor level and tenure is awarded during your seventh year of an academic appointment. If you are not on a tenure track appointment, making a 6-year plan allows you to think about how your current position fits into your long-term goals.

However, you should think beyond 6 years. What are your overall career goals? Yes, those goals may change along the way, but having some preliminary goals helps you to focus your efforts.

Navigating your career is never a solo effort. McKinney (2010) suggested that being a faculty member is like being a juggler. Planning carefully will help you manage this juggling act and facilitate career success. In many academic organizations, you submit your tenure dossier in your sixth year. In addition, those who have nontenure track positions may also have to submit dossiers as part of an evaluation or promotion process. Therefore, part of career success is planning for dossier submission on the first day of your new academic appointment.

The purpose of this chapter is to present strategies for your career development and help you to think not only about the tenure benchmark but also long term about your future career directions. You will learn how to capitalize on available resources that will help you achieve a satisfying career. Moreover, you will learn specific strategies that will help you in preparing for promotion and tenure, or for continued reappointment in institutions where tenure is not an option. You will also learn strategies for more long-term career planning.

PATHWAYS TO CAREER LONGEVITY

Several types of academic appointments exist. The majority of universities and colleges have traditional tenure track appointments. Some academic institutions have clinical appointments, which may or may not be considered a type of tenure track appointment. Other institutions have year-to-year appointments or multiyear renewable contracts.

The Traditional Tenure Track Appointment

Academic tenure is predicated on the notion of academic freedom and economic freedom found in what is sometimes called the "Red Book" published by the American Association of University Professors (AAUP; 2006). In 1940, the AAUP formulated the "Statement of Principles on Academic Freedom and Tenure" (AAUP, p. 3). This statement has formed the basis for how tenure is enacted in institutions of higher learning. According to this statement, faculty have the freedom to do research and publish the results and have freedom of speech related to the subject matter being taught. However, the AAUP states that "it is improper . . . to fail to present the subject matter of the course as announced to the students and as approved by the faculty in their collective responsibility for the curriculum" (p. 174). In other words, a faculty member has an obligation to include content that is prescribed by the curriculum and the individual course syllabi. If you are teaching an adult health class that focuses on cardiovascular disease, you cannot decide to teach only about orthopedics. You can, however, choose what paradigm cases should be presented to illustrate the course concepts. You also are free to choose appropriate teaching strategies as long as you can demonstrate learning outcomes.

Criticizing institutional and program policies is also considered protected speech (Finkin, 1988). If you criticize policies, you need to be mindful of how you present your views. Although most tenure documents do not specifically list being a good colleague as essential for achieving tenure, being a good academic colleague does factor into tenure decisions. Tenure committees might not favorably view a person who complains all the time, even with good teaching evaluations and productive scholarship record.

Freedom of speech also extends to your choice of a scholarship agenda. However, this freedom is tempered by the fact that some organizations require securing grant funds to achieve tenure. If your scholarship agenda does not garner grant funding, then you might want to reconsider your scholarly focus. In addition, your chosen area of scholarship needs to be one that is a good "fit" for the mission of the institution and program. For example, if your university stresses the scholarship of discovery and you are more interested in the scholarship of teaching, personnel committees may not consider favorably your scholarly productivity in any retention, tenure, and promotion decisions.

The AAUP (2006) statement goes on to say that as private citizens, faculty have complete freedom of speech. However, faculty should know that members of the public might view them as representatives of the academic institution. Therefore, faculty members should attempt to show respect for the institution by tempering critique of the employing institution in public forums, such as letters to the editor in the local newspapers.

With regard to economic security, once tenure has been achieved, the AAUP says faculty should expect continuous employment. However, an educational institution can dismiss a faculty member for financial reasons, or for just cause, usually inappropriate behavior, or failing to duly perform assigned duties, such as not showing up for classes.

The initial traditional tenure track appointment for a new faculty member is usually at the assistant professor level. In exceptional cases, you might be appointed at a rank higher than assistant professor. However, such cases are usually reserved for experienced faculty who are specifically recruited for their well-established expertise.

In most institutions, it takes 7 years for tenure to be awarded, with the decision being made in the sixth year of employment. If you have had teaching experience prior to your current position, your prospective employer may offer you years of credit toward tenure. Typically, you might be offered 1 to 3 years' credit. Consequently, you may be evaluated for tenure as early as your third year of employment. If you have a strong record of service, scholarship, and teaching, you might be in good shape for tenure, provided that you have continued on the same productive trajectory that you demonstrated in your previous position. Generally, however, unless you have a very strong record, accepting a shortened time before going for tenure could put you in jeopardy for not achieving this important career benchmark.

When planning your journey toward tenure, keep in mind that review committees want to see results of your efforts across the spectrum of scholarship, teaching, and service. With that in mind, make sure that with regard to scholarship you will have demonstrable products at least by the third year of employment and certainly by the tenure decision. Those products must be similar to the requirements outlined in departmental tenure documents. If the departmental criteria emphasize grants and peer-reviewed journal articles, the committee may not give much weight to book chapters and non-peer-reviewed articles when the committee makes its decision regarding your tenure. Tenure criteria may speak to the need for establishing a national reputation. Therefore, in the tenure decision process, personnel committees probably will give less weight to presentations at the local and state levels and more weight to national and international presentations.

If the criteria speak to professional leadership, then mere organizational membership will not count. Neither will participation in a community band sponsored by a parks and recreation department count toward service. Refer back to Chapter 7 for a more thorough discussion regarding your service requirements.

As mentioned throughout this text, your place of employment influences tenure requirements. Community colleges will have a heavy emphasis upon the scholarship of teaching and service, whereas nursing programs located in academic health sciences centers more than likely will place more weight upon the scholarship of discovery (traditional research). Seek out members of review committees for advice on how to make sure you are on track toward tenure. Your program administrator can also assist you in planning for that all important tenure decision.

Important Milestones Along the Pathway to Tenure

The tenure decision is not a one-time decision. You must achieve certain benchmarks along the way. According to AAUP guidelines, during the first year of your probationary period, you must be notified by March 1 if your appointment will not be renewed. If non-reappointment occurs during the second year, the institution must notify you by December 15. Beginning in the third year, you must be given 1 year's notice of nonrenewal (AAUP, 2006). Given that fact, many institutions view your third year review as critical to your success. Review committees at this juncture will try to give you a thorough assessment of your strengths in teaching, research, and service. At the same time, the committee should give you an indication if any improvements are needed.

Some organizations have a conditional reappointment category. This type of reappointment usually means that review committees believe that you have the potential to achieve tenure if you meet the conditions set forth for reappointment, such as producing additional publications or improving your teaching. Unless service is highly valued, as in the case of community engagement, rarely is minimal service cause for conditional reappointment or nonrenewal. If you do not meet the conditions of your reappointment the following year, then the personnel committee will recommend non reappointment notification. Nonrenewal at the third year or beyond means that you have not demonstrated that you can produce what is necessary to achieve tenure.

Sometimes your progress toward tenure might be altered for family responsibilities. Some faculty will use the provisions of the Family Medical Leave Act to care for newborns or elders in their family. Furthermore, many institutions allow faculty members to lengthen the "tenure clock" because of parenting or elder care responsibilities or personal illness or health problems. The time to tenure is not indefinite, but adding 1 to 2 years to the usual pretenure time is not unheard of. While these provisions are available to faculty, many choose not to use them for fear of adverse consequences such as a negative tenure decision (Wolf-Wendel & Ward, 2006). If you are one who might need additional time on the tenure clock because of family responsibilities or other issues that might interfere with your productivity, become familiar with your institution's written policies. You might also talk with peers about how your department views these policies. An affirmative action officer can also guide you if you feel that these policies are not available to you, even though they exist in written form. You might have to be assertive in advocating for your rights as defined under these policies.

Decisions regarding tenure are often linked with promotion. Some institutions do not grant tenure at the assistant professor level. In other words, if you are not promoted to associate professor, you do not achieve tenure. Other institutions, primarily those who have a strong teaching focus and modest scholarship requirements, do grant tenure in the rank of assistant professor. Such cases are often reserved for outstanding teachers who have little scholarly productivity, but strong professional service.

Think About . . .

What do the program and institution expect of me in teaching, research, and service as I work toward tenure? Where should I focus my efforts?

Levels of Review

Who is involved in your reappointment and tenure decisions varies with the institution. In the majority of cases, a committee of your colleagues plays a major role in your tenure decision. Depending upon the organizational structure, your department chair, departmental personnel committee, school or college personnel (promotion and tenure) committee, and dean may make independent decisions regarding reappointment, tenure, and promotion. In cases where the nursing program exists in a nondepartmentalized school, the all-school committee, followed by the dean or director, makes the initial recommendations for reappointment, tenure, and promotion.

Once the decisions are made at the school or college level, some organizations have an all-university committee that also makes a tenure recommendation, followed by the chief academic officer and the president. Some places also require the board of trustees to affirm tenure and promotion decisions. At other institutions, no all-university committee exists. Decisions made at the school or college level go directly to the institution's chief academic officer and then on to the president and board of trustees.

In addition to the internal levels of review, some academic organizations require that external reviewers make recommendations regarding whether you should receive tenure and promotion. Prior to internal reviews, your department or program might solicit academic experts in your field to review your tenure and promotion dossier. In some cases, you could be asked to submit a list of experts from which your organization can choose. Your organization sends your materials to these reviewers. Reviewers will make statements regarding the strength of your teaching, scholarship, or service. Their reviews will then become a part of your dossier reviewed by internal committees. In some cases, these external reviews are confidential and in other cases, by law, you can have access to the external reviewers' comments.

Jill—Path to Tenure

Jill is a faculty member at a regional state university. Prior to coming to academe, she was a clinical specialist in an intensive care unit at a hospital in an academic health sciences center. Her interest in teaching was sparked by being a preceptor for undergraduate nursing students.

In her first year, Jill taught in a senior-level adult health course. During that time, she became acquainted with the course and participated in a team that delivered the didactic course material in a classroom setting. Teaching was a bit harder than she had imagined, but she persevered and at the end of the first year, she felt more comfortable in her teaching role. In addition to her teaching, she worked to write a grant to continue her doctoral research concerned with preventing hospital readmissions for patients with congestive heart failure. In the process of writing her grant, she was able to develop a network of supportive colleagues. She also was able to present the findings from her dissertation at a national meeting.

At the end of the first year, she met with her department chair to review her accomplishments. Her chair commended her for her work, but reminded Jill that she needed to have at least one article in press by the end of the next academic year and further develop her scholarly productivity. Following her grant submission, Jill spent the summer writing, and by the beginning of the next academic year she had two articles submitted for publication. Both were accepted. Although her grant was not funded, through the network she had established she was able to be a part of another grant submission team and this time the grant was funded.

By her third year, Jill was teaching in both the undergraduate and graduate programs, she had two articles in peer-reviewed journals, one book chapter in a major textbook, and was a coinvestigator on a major grant. She had participated on one nursing program committee. By the

(continued)

time she submitted her tenure dossier in her sixth year, she had five peer-reviewed articles, four national presentations, and had another grant funded—this time she was the principal investigator. Also, she had chaired a nursing program committee and also was on a university committee, and had chaired a national taskforce. As expected, she was promoted to associate professor and was tenured.

Jill's story in Case Study 8.1 illustrates a traditional path toward tenure. When considering Jill's case, notice how she uses her yearly evaluations to improve her performance and ensure her success when she applies for tenure and promotion to associate professor. What can you learn from Jill's case as you consider your own pathway toward tenure?

Inherent in the reappointment, promotion, and tenure decision process is the ability for faculty to appeal a negative decision. If you should receive a negative review followed by a terminal contract, know your due process rights. Your faculty handbook should outline the procedures for appeal. In most cases, negative reviews are rarely a surprise. Your yearly reviews up until the point of nonreappointment or tenure denial should have given you an honest appraisal of your progress toward tenure. Closely following the advice given in these reviews should set you on a solid course for success when it comes to the tenure decision.

Tenure and reappointment denials are rare, but do happen. Sometimes budgetary constraints prohibit institutions from awarding tenure. On the other hand, if you are teaching in a graduate program and the faculty eliminate the specialty in which you have been teaching, you might not get tenure because the program has been eliminated and there is not a fit for your expertise.

Alternative Academic Pathways

Not all academic appointments are traditional tenure track appointments. Many institutions now have clinical track appointments. Those hired on clinical tracks may not always have the terminal degrees that are required for most traditional tenure track appointments. Nevertheless, they are hired because their clinical expertise is a recognized asset, particularly in the education of prelicensure students (Lee, Kim, Roh, Shin, & Kim, 2007). However, many institutions now require terminal degrees, such as the Doctorate of Nursing Practice, even for clinical appointments.

Most state boards of nursing and accreditation agencies require that the majority of clinical faculty have a minimum of a master's degree. Clinical faculty may be hired full-time or part-time. Some may have joint appointments with clinical agencies. Their duties include clinical teaching and in many instances classroom teaching as well.

Whether clinical appointments are on a tenure track is variable. If the appointments are on a tenure track, requirements for achieving tenure will differ somewhat from the requirements for faculty with traditional tenure track appointments. The major difference is usually the scholarship requirement. If the clinical tenure track requirements include publications, these publications will most often focus on the scholarship of teaching and application, rather than the scholarship of discovery (see Chapters 5, 6, and 7). Clinical track appointments may also have heavier professional service requirements. One advantage to the institution is that clinical faculty are often preferred by students, who view them as more in touch with the realities of the practice environment than tenure track faculty, who may not have an active clinical practice (Lee et al., 2007).

Clinical faculty may also be employed part-time or on year-to-year contracts or renewable multiyear contracts. Such employment arrangements allow the institution the ability to control faculty numbers based on fluctuating student enrollments.

In some instances, clinical faculty, not on tenure track appointments, may still be eligible for promotions. Such faculty submit materials, just like tenure track faculty, for personnel committees to evaluate for promotion. Institutional promotion criteria are likely to be similar to the criteria at institutions that do have clinical tenure track appointments. Promotion opportunities reflect the importance of clinical teaching in nursing and other professional programs.

Some clinical faculty with young children might prefer part-time arrangements or year-to-year appointments as these arrangements allow them flexibility when caring for family members. Other faculty who are in doctoral programs might also prefer part-time options as well.

Documenting Your Accomplishments

No matter what type of employment contract you have, you will be expected to present evidence of your effectiveness as a faculty member. How and when you submit your materials will vary according to your type of employment. Faculty on the traditional tenure track or the clinical tenure track may be required to submit yearly a dossier that documents progress toward the tenure decision. If yearly submissions are not required, you should still collect evidence of your accomplishments from the first day of your employment. In cases where faculty do not submit yearly dossiers, faculty should be prepared to submit dossiers in their third year of employment, at the time when the tenure decision is made, and for the times when promotion occurs beyond tenure. Institutions that employ faculty who work on full- or part-time yearly contracts may also require those faculty to submit a formal dossier in hard copy or online.

In many institutions, all faculty, tenured or not, prepare yearly faculty activity reports and submit them online or in hard copy. The annual reports often include a current vita and perhaps a list of accomplishments achieved in teaching, scholarship, and service during the current academic or calendar year. These reports, which are not as in depth as dossiers, are used to document individual, program, and school or college productivity. In an era when stakeholders such as legislators, boards of trustees, and donors want evidence that their investments in educational institutions are wise, documentation of faculty productivity must be readily available. These annual reports may be in addition to formal dossiers used for pretenure evaluations and promotion decisions. These reports may, in some cases, be used for merit pay decisions for all, including those on the tenure track or not.

Exhibit 8.1 shows what materials should be included in your dossier. You must collect relevant documents and keep them in an organized fashion so that you can easily retrieve them when you present your materials. A good strategy is to place the documents in a separate folder for each year. You might write on the outside of the folder "committee assignments," "teaching loads," and other titles that can help you organize your materials. On the other hand, you might prepare a table of contents for the folder or you may arrange your materials in the folder according to accomplishments in teaching, scholarship, and service. That way, when you prepare your yearly evaluation materials and the tenure or promotion dossier, you will have all your materials organized. Of course, computer backup ensures that you do not lose important items you might want to include in your dossier. Having all your important documents in alternate forms prevents the loss of materials, either through hard drive failure or some catastrophe that ruins hard copy documents.

Exhibit 8.1

Evidence for Retention, Tenure, and Promotion Dossiers

Items That Document Your Teaching Role

1. Syllabi
2. Copies of Web-based and other course materials
3. Tests
4. Examples of student assignments
5. Examples of publications resulting from student assignments
6. Peer evaluations
7. Student evaluations
8. Certificates from relevant continuing education

Items That Document Your Scholarship Role

1. Copies of articles, book chapters, book cover pages
2. Grants (funded and unfunded)
3. Conference proceedings
4. Conference abstracts
5. Letters of acceptance for not-yet-published works
6. Copies of CDs, software, or links to Web pages

Items That Document Your Service Role

1. Copies of committee minutes
2. Letters acknowledging service
3. Documentation of leadership in professional or campus organizations
4. Clinical practice contracts

Some institutions or departments have very specific requirements with regard to dossier preparation, including the maximum number of pages the dossier should contain. Other institutions and departments leave what to include more open. In all cases, however, the goal of the dossier is to "sell yourself" in an accurate manner. What follows are suggestions for a dossier that is submitted in hard copy in an organization with open guidelines for dossier preparation. If your institution uses an e-portfolio, you will need to follow those guidelines for electronic submission.

Those who review your documents should be able to locate your materials easily. A table of contents is always a good idea, as are dividers with typed labels. The dividers separate out evidence for teaching, scholarship, and service. Remember, this is a professional document, so the cover should be plain.

Usually, you should place a current vita in the front of the dossier. However, be sure and find out what format your institution requires. (Refer to the discussion and exhibit in Chapter 3 that outline the differences between a vita and resume.) Most institutions suggest that you precede each section of your dossier with a statement that summarizes your accomplishments in a particular area. For example, before the section relevant to teaching, you should include your philosophy of teaching. Review committees look for how you reflect upon your strengths as a teacher and how you use your challenges to improve your teaching. For instance, you might be very strong in the use of media, but need more work on using active learning strategies in your classroom. Therefore, you could mention what you are doing to increase the use of more active learning in your didactic teaching. Reflecting upon your student and peer evaluations, which you should include in your dossier, also shows that you use the critical appraisal of your teaching to improve your course delivery.

Student and peer evaluations from year to year should provide evidence that you are improving as a teacher. All experienced teachers have, from time to time, student evaluations that are not very good. If that happens to you, yes, you must include these evaluations in your dossier. However, in your teaching statement reflect upon what might have gone wrong. For example, you might have tried something new in your course delivery that did not work. Your teaching statement would then show why you think the new strategy was not effective and how you used student feedback to improve your course delivery. By doing so, you show that you are committed to excellence in teaching. Whether you include any student thank you notes is up to you. However, your course evaluations, peer reviews, syllabi and other course materials, and teaching statement should be sufficient to demonstrate your teaching effectiveness.

Since some faculty who evaluate your dossier will likely not be nurses, you should make the case that your scholarly work is rigorous. Faculty from outside of the nursing discipline may not understand the nature of professional publications and the demands of the clinical teaching environment. Your reflective statements included in your dossier should explain why your accomplishments are of value. For example, if you did a major course redesign that included new teaching strategies that you systematically evaluated, you could show how the redesign positively affected student learning outcomes.

Even your nurse colleagues, who have a different expertise from yourself, may not be familiar with your publication and presentation venues. Therefore, in some way, you should designate which of the conferences and journals listed in your dossier are peer reviewed. You may also have to state the impact factor of journals in which you have published. An impact factor reflects a journal's quality as evidenced by the number of times articles published in that journal in a particular year are cited by others who publish in other journals (Thomson Reuters, 2010).

In your statements, highlight how your work is aligned with your university's and nursing program's mission and strategic goals. For instance, if your university stresses service learning, in your teaching and service statements, identify which student activities can be categorized as service learning. If grant writing is stressed, under your statement regarding your scholarship highlight your grant activities.

Pretenure faculty often ask, "How much material should be retained year to year?" You should seek guidance from your department chair and members of the review committees. Some institutions and committees want everything retained from year to year and some want only selected materials retained, such as publications and course evaluations.

When you submit your dossier for tenure and promotion, your narratives should emphasize your growth as a scholar, teacher, and nursing professional. A current curriculum vitae will show all the activities you have participated in during your previous years on faculty. Each of your three sections of your dossier should include a compilation of all your activities. However, seek guidance from those who will review your dossier regarding whether all materials from prior years should be included. Some institutions have strict requirements regarding how much documentation should be included in a tenure and promotion dossier.

With regard to teaching, one way to demonstrate your progress is to develop graphs that show the quantitative ratings of your teaching. Examples of your current syllabi should be sufficient. Also, include any innovative teaching materials that you have developed. In addition to the items suggested in Exhibit 8.1, your statement that highlights your scholarship accomplishments should reflect how your scholarship has developed with regard to focus.

If your review committees stress validation of service contributions, you might solicit letters from organizations where you have provided service. Furthermore, if it is the culture of your institution to do so, you could solicit letters from professional colleagues who support your quest for tenure and promotion.

Do not hesitate to show your strengths. At the same time, do not exaggerate. Any information that you present that is not accurate could be cause for tenure denial. Above all, preparing materials for tenure and promotion involves selling your accomplishments in the best and most accurate way, while demonstrating your potential for future contributions to the institution and the profession.

Think About . . .

Who will be reading my dossier? How can I prepare my dossier so that I present myself in the best light?

Posttenure Review

Once you achieve tenure, either through a traditional tenure track or through a clinical track, you may still have to verify your continued worth to the institution or you may have to submit materials for merit pay reviews. Increasingly, stakeholders want evidence that all faculty are productive. According to Neal (2008), one goal of posttenure review is to promote professional development. Ideally, tenured faculty would look at these reviews as a way to continually evaluate performance and use the reviews to set goals for performance improvement. Despite some concern by the AAUP that posttenure review is a threat to academic freedom, Hawkins, Graham, and Hall (2007) stated that an institution can use posttenure reviews to not only promote performance improvement but also celebrate and reward excellence. Posttenure review is here to stay, so you will need to carry forth skills you learned in preparing materials for pretenure evaluations throughout your career.

Another reason to continue documenting your accomplishments is for such things as institutional teaching awards. As you get further along in your career, you may use the documentation to substantiate nominations for regional and national awards.

CHARTING YOUR COURSE FOR SUCCESS

Most likely, your immediate concerns revolve around the reappointment, tenure, and promotion processes. However, these processes are just a reflection of achieving your short- and long-term goals. Setting reasonable year-to-year goals, as well as longer term goals, helps you to focus your efforts. As you have learned throughout this book, finding ways to use your time wisely will help you achieve success. Make the most of your professional network. When you go to meetings, forge relationships with persons who can help you with your scholarship. For example, if you hear a presentation on a topic of interest, the presenter could perhaps serve as a consultant on a grant that you write.

Postdoctoral Education

Short-term and long-term goals are not divorced from each other. You, of course, cannot achieve long-term success without meeting benchmarks along the way. One opportunity to consider if your goal is to develop as a researcher with a solid research agenda is the role of postdoctoral education in your career. Postdoctoral education has long been a hallmark of academic careers in the hard sciences. More recently, postdoctoral education has gained prominence in nursing education (Montgomery, Semenic, & Edwards, 2008). The focus of postdoctoral education is to develop independent skills in grant writing and research. Several models exist. The traditional postdoctoral fellowship consists of 1 to 2 years of intense research and grant writing at a university where experienced researchers can mentor you and help you gain expertise beyond what you gained in your doctoral education. Another model involves a combination of intense on-site work at a major university combined with work done at your employing institution (Gennaro, Deatrick, Dobal, Jemmott, & Ball, 2007). In this model, faculty who are place bound have access to mentors who assist them in developing skills that in the short term help them achieve tenure at their home institution, and at the same time set them up for a long-term research career.

The Role of Mentors in Your Career

Mentors are important to your career development. The National League for Nursing (NLN), in fact, has published a position statement recognizing the critical role of mentors in retaining nursing faculty in the workforce (NLN, 2006). In the traditional mentorship relationship, a single mentor hooks up with a protégé, and through a sustained relationship, the protégé grows and develops in his or her career.

Other models, however, may be more suited to academe. Building a network of mentors that can help you during various phases of your career may be more beneficial than having just one mentor (Sorcinelli & Yun, 2007; Washburn, 2007). You might have, in your early career, mentors who assist you with your teaching and another group of mentors who assist you with your research agenda. Others may help you develop your leadership skills in professional organizations.

You might ask, "How do I find experienced faculty to mentor me?" One place to start is in your own department. Ask an experienced faculty to sit in on your classes and critique your presentations. If your teaching is online, have a person who is an expert in distance education comment upon your course sites. Teaching mentors are especially important if you have had little experience in teaching, as well as little formal nursing education coursework.

Some institutions have extensive faculty orientation programs. Forge relationships with presenters in those programs. Even if the presenters are outside your department, they can help you learn how to navigate the academic environment.

Your own department is a good place to start for help with research. However, experts in your field may well be outside your department or even your institution. You can meet these people at meetings. Staff research and grant offices at your institution often give classes on grant writing. Faculty outside your department may have methodological expertise that you need to get a program of research started. Besides, interprofessional research teams often have a better chance of garnering grants than do single disciplinary teams.

Your peers may also serve as mentors (Jacelon, Zucker, Staccarini, & Henneman, 2003). Junior faculty can share knowledge learned in doctoral programs, form support networks, and develop joint programs of scholarship.

Mentors are not just for beginning faculty. As you progress in your career, you may need different mentors to help you advance (NLN, 2006). For example, if you have developed leadership skills at the local, state, and regional levels, you might need different mentors to help you become a leader at the national or international level. As you become more comfortable in your teaching role, you may need mentors who will help you learn new teaching methodologies.

Mentors are important, so develop your network. Having support throughout your career will help you develop into an independent, seasoned faculty member.

A View to the Future

When you begin a new job in academe, feelings of uncertainty could overwhelm you. However, writing down your goals and placing them in a safe place for frequent review can help you stay focused. Set goals for each academic year as well as what you want to achieve 5, 10, and even 15 years from now. For example, more short-term goals may include receiving a major grant by your third year on the tenure track and publishing one peer-reviewed article per year. For a more long-term goal, you may state that you want to be a department chair within 10 years of beginning a new faculty position. This does not mean that your goals are static and can never change. Nevertheless, setting short- and long-term goals keeps you from feeling as if you have no control over your career. Table 8.1 shows an example of career goals for a faculty member at a regional state university.

Think About . . .

What are your career goals? Would you be willing to move to achieve those goals or will you match your goals to what is available at your current institution?

TABLE 8.1 Setting Goals

Ruth, a new faculty member in a regional state university, has set the following goals:

TYPE OF GOAL	TEACHING	SCHOLARSHIP	SERVICE
1-year	Become familiar with courses and develop teaching materials	Publish results of dissertation Make one regional presentation	Serve on one program curriculum committee Seek peer reviewer opportunities
3-year	Revise course materials to include heavy service learning component Begin work on interprofessional education within the health professions Begin teaching in the graduate program in nursing education	Receive grant to support scholarship of teaching Total national presentations = 2	Chair one program curriculum committee Member of one institutional curriculum committee
6-year	Have health professions interprofessional course in place	Have a total of four articles in peer-reviewed nursing education journals and a total of four national presentations	Member of one national committee in professional organization related to teaching Chair one institutional committee Consult on interprofessional education
10-year	Program chair of graduate program in nursing education	Established reputation as expert in interprofessional education	Elected leadership position in nursing education professional organization

To Move or Not to Move: That Is the Question

One question arises when you begin to consider your career pathway: "Should I plan on staying at the same academic institution for my entire career?" The answer to this question is not as easy as you may think. One factor that will help determine whether you consider moving is your overall career goals. If you want to move into academic administration, you may have to move unless internal opportunities exist. Even if you can move into administration at your current institution, you may be more successful at another institution because, in some cases, friendship relationships may interfere with your ability to make decisions that are in the best interests of the academic unit.

Moving forward with your research agenda may also prompt a move. Sometimes you might need a different level of support than what is available at your current place of employment to fully achieve your research goals.

Personal factors also influence whether you consider moving. You may need to take into account family considerations. Is your spouse or partner willing to move? Do you have children who have special needs that require special services? Being creative in your thinking, however, may allow you to take advantage of an opportunity at another academic institution. With the advent of telecommuting, many faculty find that they can change jobs with little family disruption.

Moving does advance your career. However, moves at certain points in your career can send a problematic message to a prospective employer. If you move in your fourth or fifth year of employment in a faculty position, another employer might view this move as a way to avoid tenure denial. If you move too often, without explanation, future employers may question your investment in an institution.

Case Study 8.2 illustrates the decision process used in setting and achieving career goals. Notice how Tom starts out with one set of goals and then as one opportunity comes along he reconsiders his long-term goals. Would you make the same decisions as Tom?

THE WORLD IS YOURS

A nursing faculty career is one of the most rewarding paths you can take in the nursing profession. With the faculty shortage that exists now and for the future, embarking on a faculty career is a worthy

Case Study 8.2

Tom—A Career Path Changed

Tom has taught in an associate degree nursing program. He really enjoyed teaching and thought he would be satisfied teaching for the rest of his career. One year his program director resigned and he was appointed interim program chair. He found that he liked academic administration, but realized he needed more education if he were to serve in an administrative role during his career. He stepped down from his interim chair position, but continued to teach while he was enrolled in a doctoral program where he majored in nursing education and had a minor in academic leadership. Following graduation, he decided to stay in his current position because of family considerations and await the opportunity to move into a permanent academic administrative role at his place of employment. Within a few years, the program director position became open and he applied for this position. Tom was chosen to be the nursing program chair. However, after 4 years as program director, Tom decided that his heart was really in full-time teaching. He stepped down from the director position, because he wanted to seek another career challenge. He decided to apply for teaching positions within a university setting. He was hired at a university not far from where he lived.

endeavor. The path you forge will inevitably have bumps along the way. However, use these challenges as opportunities for growth. You can determine your own road for success and have the opportunity to facilitate the learning of future nurses, advance the discipline of nursing, and provide leadership within the profession. By doing so, you will have a long and fulfilling career.

Opportunities for Further Reflection
1. How will you handle the challenges in your career?
2. What might cause you to change your career goals?

REFERENCES

American Association of University Professors. (2006). *AAUP policy documents & reports* (10th ed.). Washington, DC: Author.

Finkin, M. W. (1988). The tenure system. In L. A. Deneef, C. D. Goodwin, & E. S. McCrate (Eds.), *The academic's handbook* (pp. 86–100). Durham, NC: Duke University Press.

Gennaro, S., Deatrick, J. A., Dobal, M. T., Jemmott, L. S., & Ball, K. R. (2007). An alternative model for postdoctoral education of nurses engaged in research with potentially vulnerable populations. *Nursing Outlook, 55*(6), 275–281.

Hawkins, A. G. Jr., Graham, R. D., & Hall, R. F. (2007). Tenure as a fact of academic life: A methodology for managing the performance of tenured professors. *Education and the Law, 19*(1), 41–57.

Jacelon, C. S., Zucker, D. M., Staccarini, J. M., & Henneman, E. A. (2003). Peer mentoring for tenure-track faculty. *Journal of Professional Nursing, 19*(6), 335–338.

Lee, W. H., Kim, C. J., Roh, Y. S., Shin, H., & Kim, M. J. (2007). Clinical track faculty: Merits and issues. *Journal of Professional Nursing, 23*(1), 5–12.

McKinney, M. (2010). *Becoming a successful academic takes more than intelligence.* Retrieved May 31, 2010, from http://www.successfulacademic.com/index.htm

Montgomery, P., Semenic, S., & Edwards, E., (2008). Post-doctoral training in nursing: A consideration of opportunities and strategies. *Canadian Journal of Nursing Leadership, 21*(1), 36–43.

National League for Nursing. (2006). Statement: Mentoring new faculty. *Nursing Education Perspectives, 27*(2), 110–113.

Neal, A. D. (2008). Reviewing post-tenure review. *Academe, 94*(5), 27–30.

Sorcinelli, M. D., & Yun, J. (2007). From mentor to mentoring networks: Mentoring in the new academe. *Change, 39*(6), 58–61.

Thomson Reuters. (2010). *The Thomson Reuters impact factor.* Retrieved May 31, 2010, from http://thomsonreuters.com/products_services/science/free/essays/impact_factor/

Washburn, M. H. (2007). Mentoring women faculty: An instrumental case study of strategic collaboration. *Mentoring & Teaching, 15*(1), 57–72.

Wolf-Wendel, L. E., & Ward, K. (2006). Academic life and motherhood: Variations by institutional types. *Higher Education, 52*(3), 487–521.

Afterword

We have shared with you our advice for a long and rewarding career as a nursing faculty member. We hope you will consider what we have to say and use what makes sense to you and your career pathway. Our career narratives have informed the advice we have shared with you. Therefore, what follows are our stories so that you can see how we arrived at the career guidance we have shared.

BETSY FRANK

I always knew I wanted to be a nurse. When I graduated high school, my parents insisted I go to a baccalaureate program, despite the fact that the majority of nursing education in the late 1960s was at the diploma level. During my undergraduate days, my professors challenged me to think about my career goals. As a sophomore nursing student, I read an article in the *American Journal of Nursing* by Frances Reiter (1966). She wrote about a master's-prepared clinical nurse specialist. I remember thinking, "Aha! That is what I want to do." I immediately planned to continue my education. After graduation from The Ohio State University and getting married, my husband and I moved to Seattle, where I enrolled in the master's program at the University of Washington School of Nursing. I was able to combine an interest in advanced clinical practice and nursing education. One of my mentors there told me to keep a file of research ideas and use them to build my research career. I did that and used the folder as a springboard for later work. My professors in my master's program instilled within me an understanding of the importance of publishing and becoming engaged in all aspects of the academic role. I completed my master's degree within 2 years of graduating from my baccalaureate degree.

My husband joined the Air Force, and we began 23 years of traveling. Yes, I based Elizabeth in Chapter 3 on my career. My first job post master's was in education. Throughout the time my husband was in the Air Force, I worked in a variety of jobs, including being a nurse clinician/nursing supervisor and teaching in associate degree, baccalaureate, and master's programs. We had two daughters along the way, and I was able to obtain my PhD in educational administration at the University of Utah.

I chose my doctoral education pathway because after being an administrator of a small associate degree program I thought I wanted to be a dean. I focused my course work and dissertation on that goal. With moving and time off for child rearing, I graduated from my doctoral program 12 years after getting my master's degree.

Following graduation from my doctoral program, I taught at Wright State University for 4 years before moving to Spain for 3 years. Even there, I was able to do nursing workshops and teach a research course in a non-nursing master's program. Perhaps the best part of the time overseas (aside from the travel of course) was the think time. Where did I want my career to go when my husband retired from the military? I knew that I wanted a regional university where I could develop a program of scholarship but also focus on teaching. When we returned from overseas, I was able to teach again in a bachelor and master's program like I had at Wright State University, this time at the University of New Mexico.

During these more than 20 years, I learned that I could combine career and parenthood, even with a husband in the military. I had to build a support network wherever I went, which helped me when needed. And, yes, multitasking did work! The advice I gave in Chapter 4 to work on your class preparation or other academic responsibilities while children do homework was effective.

Then the time came. My husband retired from the Air Force, and we chose to relocate closer to our homes so we could help care for aging parents. I began a long career as a faculty member at a regional state university, Indiana State University. I was a department chair for 6 years and decided that I really wanted to teach full-time, rather than continue on the academic administration career pathway. Surprisingly so, I learned I loved to teach online. I found I could be just as interactive as I was in the classroom.

Each place I worked I capitalized on my opportunities. I published, was active in professional organizations, and built my professional network. Looking back, I know the ability to profit from my varied opportunities has lent to the richness of my career.

As I approach retirement from full-time teaching, I know that I will never totally disengage from nursing education. I will continue to teach part-time and remain active in professional organizations. However, I will have more time for other pursuits.

What did I learn from a career pathway that, in retrospect, was not totally planned? I learned that you can plan long term, but when circumstances change, pause and reevaluate. When I entered my master's program, I thought that was as far as I would go. However, several of my professors in my master's program planted the seeds for doctoral education. I grew in my role as an educator through my exposure to a variety of educational settings and through a variety of mentors along the way. I learned that each place we are in life has things to teach and help us grow. Most of all, I learned that nursing education is my passion. As an educator, I take great satisfaction from seeing students I have taught achieve great things. I hope all of you will discover your passion in nursing education as well.

JUDY HALSTEAD

Like my colleague Betsy, I also knew that I always wanted to be a nurse. The problem for me was I also always wanted to be a teacher. As a young child, I vividly recall spending many hours lining all my dolls up on the living room couch. In my play world they were either "going to school" or "in the hospital." At the time, I didn't realize that my pathway toward a career in nursing education had already had its beginning!

When the time came to make a choice about college, after much thought, I chose to go to nursing school—after all, nurses always have a job, don't they? After having spent 4 years as a Candy Striper in the local hospital, I already knew that I enjoyed the hospital atmosphere, and working alongside the RNs caring for people had convinced me that I would enjoy a nursing career. Again, just like my colleague Betsy's experience, my parents insisted that I go to college and get my baccalaureate degree.

I enrolled in the University of Evansville for my undergraduate degree. As a senior nursing student, I found that as much as I enjoyed caring for my patients, I also spent a considerable amount of my time during my clinical experiences watching my instructors in their interactions with students. Somewhere in my last semester of undergraduate education, a light bulb came on for me, and I realized that I did not have to make a choice between a career in nursing or teaching, after all—I could actually do both!

So when my clinical instructor asked me about my career goals in my final exit interview with her, I said, "I want to do what you do." I remember feeling a little embarrassed to admit to her that I wanted to be a nursing instructor; I was still a student with very little "real" nursing experience, and how could I possibly think that I could have a career teaching others how to be a nurse? However, my instructor did a wonderful thing in response to my nervous admission that I wanted to teach nursing—she simply said to me, "And you would be good at it." She proceeded to advise me on getting some experience as a nurse and, most importantly, to enroll in a master's degree program to prepare myself for teaching. At most, it was a 15-minute conversation, one that I am sure the faculty herself quickly forgot. However, to this day, I remember how she took me seriously and gave me my first real career advice. That was all it took to encourage me to pursue being a nurse educator at an early stage of my career, and I left her office with a career plan.

Within 3 years, I was working on my MSN (at the University of Evansville) and had my first position as a nursing instructor at Deaconess Hospital School of Nursing, a diploma school of nursing in Evansville, Indiana. I learned a great deal from my faculty mentors in that position, and for that I owe them a debt of gratitude. The faculty were some of the most dedicated and creative individuals I have ever had the good fortune with whom to work. When I left the position 8 years later to continue pursuit of my doctorate, I had developed a strong foundation in classroom teaching strategies, curriculum development, and clinical teaching skills—a foundation that has served me well for over 30 years.

I knew that if I wanted a long-term career in nursing education in a university setting, I needed to pursue a doctorate. I also knew that although I understood a great deal about clinical nursing, I did not really have an understanding of the environment in which I wished to work—higher education. With that in mind, I chose to pursue a doctorate in nursing with a major in academic administration and a minor in higher education at Indiana University School of Nursing. At the time, I had a 4-year-old son and 6-week-old daughter—and a very supportive husband! As this was before the time of distance learning (at least at the doctoral level), we relocated to Indianapolis, where I also accepted my first position to teach nursing within a university setting. It took me 15 years to progress from my BSN to my PhD, working full-time and going to school part-time.

I can honestly say that my career path in nursing education has not been a planned one, with some master plan guiding every step I have taken. The choices I have made have always been balanced by my strong connections to family. What I have done, however, is take advantage of opportunities along the way, knowing that each new experience would provide me with additional skills. Those opportunities gradually led me into academic administrative positions, where I have remained for 21 years.

In the last 30 years, my career path in nursing education has brought me into contact with more than 3,000 nursing students from whom I have learned much. It has also provided me with life-changing international nursing education experiences, a large network of faculty colleagues across the country, and the opportunity to provide national leadership within the nursing profession. I am very fortunate, indeed, that back in 1976, a nurse educator took the time to encourage me to pursue my dream—to me that is what being a nurse educator is all about.

REFERENCE

Reiter, F. (1966). The nurse-clinician. *The American Journal of Nursing, 66*(2), 274–280.

Selected Resources

These selected resources promote nursing and higher education and may provide venues for presentations and publications of nursing education research as well as resources for faculty development in the nurse educator role.

NATIONAL ORGANIZATIONS FOR HIGHER EDUCATION AND NURSING EDUCATION

American Association of University Professors (http://www.aaup .org/aaup) promotes academic freedom and shared governance in higher education. Its Collective Bargaining Congress provides resources for local collective bargaining agreements.

American Association of Colleges of Nursing (http://www.aacn.nche .edu/) is an organization that represents baccalaureate and higher degree nursing programs. AACN assists deans in promoting quality education. Position papers regarding nursing education are published as are essentials documents for bachelor's, master's, and doctoral education. AACN also provides faculty development programs where posters and papers are presented. Regular webinars are also held.

The Carnegie Foundation for the Advancement of Teaching (www .carnegiefoundation.org) promotes the development of policy and research focused on the improvement of teaching.

Commission on Collegiate Nursing Education (http://www.aacn .nche.edu/Accreditation/index.htm) accredits baccalaureate and higher degree nursing programs.

EDUCAUSE (www.educause.edu) promotes the "intelligent use of information technology in higher education" and publishes online journals, *EDUCAUSE Review* and *EDUCAUSE Quarterly*. EDUCAUSE also has a resource center and holds an annual conference.

MERLOT (http://www.merlot.org/merlot/index.htm) is the Multimedia Educational Resource for Learning and Online Teaching. This organization provides a repository of resources where faculty can upload course resources to share and likewise download teaching materials. These materials are peer reviewed by users. MERLOT also publishes the *Journal of Online Learning and Teaching* and holds an annual faculty development conference.

National League for Nursing (http://www.nln.org) promotes excellence across all levels of nursing education. The annual Faculty Summit is a venue for poster and paper presentations. Multiple faculty development programs are regularly presented around the country. The NLN regularly publishes position papers about important topics in nursing education and books about nursing education topics. The NLN sponsors the certification program for nurse educators (CNE) and the Centers for Excellence in Nursing Education. A competitive grants program funds nursing education research.

National League for Nursing Accrediting Commission, Inc. (http://www .nlnac.org/home.htm) accredits all levels of nursing education programs.

Sigma Theta Tau International (http://www.nursingsociety.org/default. aspx) is the international honor society of nursing. The biennial convention and yearly research conferences provide venues for poster and paper presentations.

REGIONAL NURSING RESEARCH SOCIETIES

The following regional research societies hold yearly conferences where posters and papers are presented. Some of these societies have nursing education research interest groups. Consult their Web pages for more information about these societies and the available conferences and publications.

Eastern Nursing Research Society (http://www.enrs-go.org/)

Midwest Nursing Research Society (http://www.mnrs.org)

Southern Nursing Research Society (http://www.snrs.org/)

Western Institute of Nursing (http://www.ohsu.edu/son/win/#)

JOURNALS AND OTHER PUBLICATIONS THAT APPEAR IN PRINT AND ONLINE

These journals and newspapers publish articles focused on nursing education and higher education.

Academe

Annual Review of Nursing Education

Chronicle of Higher Education

Computers Informatics Nursing

International Journal of Nursing Education Scholarship

Journal of Professional Nursing

Journal of Nursing Education

Nurse Educator

Nursing Outlook

Nursing Education Perspectives

BOOKS

Adams, M., & Valiga, T. (Eds.). (2009). *Achieving excellence in nursing education.* New York: National League for Nursing.

Ard, N., & Valiga, T. (Eds.). (2009). *Clinical nursing education: Current reflections.* New York: National League for Nursing.

Benner, P., Suthphen, M., Leonard, V., & Day, L. (2010). *Educating nurses: A call for radical transformation.* San Francisco: Jossey-Bass.

Billings, D. M., & Halstead, J. A. (2009). *Teaching in nursing: A guide for faculty* (3rd ed.). St. Louis, MO: Saunders Elsevier.

Bonnel, W., & Smith, K. (2010). *Teaching technologies in nursing and health professions: Beyond simulation and online courses.* New York: Springer Publishing Company.

Bradshaw, M. J., & Lowenstein, A. J. (2011). *Innovative teaching strategies in nursing and related health professions* (5th ed.). Sudbury, MA: Jones and Bartlett.

Caputi, L. (Ed.). (2010). *Teaching in nursing: An art and science* (2nd ed.). Glen Ellyn, IL: College of DuPage Press. [Note: This is a 4-volume series. Three of the volumes are in a 2nd edition.]

Fitzpatrick, J., Shultz, C., & Aiken, T. (2010). *Giving through teaching: How nurse educators are changing the world.* New York: Springer Publishing Company.

Gaberson, K. B., & Oermann, M. H. (2010). *Clinical teaching strategies in nursing* (3rd ed.). New York: Springer Publishing Company.

Halstead, J. A. (Ed.). (2007). *Nurse educator competencies: Creating an evidence-based practice for nurse educators.* New York: National League for Nursing.

Jeffries, P. (Ed.). (2007). *Simulation in nursing education: From conceptualization to evaluation.* New York: National League for Nursing.

Oermann, M. H. (2009). *Evaluation and testing in nursing education* (3rd ed.). New York: Springer Publishing Company.

Oermann, M. H., & Hays, J. C. (2010). *Writing for publication in nursing* (2nd ed.). New York: Springer Publishing Company.

Shultz, C. M. (Ed.). (2009). *Building a science of nursing education.* New York: National League for Nursing.

LISTSERVS

Nursing Education is a listserv where faculty can post questions and receive answers from colleagues around the world. Subscribe at: http://lists.uvic.ca/mailman/listinfo/nrsinged

Tomorrow's Professor is a listserv that sends out higher education faculty development postings, many of which are aimed at novice faculty. Subscribe at: https://mailman.stanford.edu/mailman/listinfo/tomorrows-professor

Index